AGE-PROOF

Beauty Alternatives You Need to Know!

by Louisa Graves

Cover Design: Hunter Business Forms Inc. Print & Promotion, Hamilton, Ontario, Canada

Illustrations: Shannon Cody Design, Los Angeles, CA.

Photographs: Babak Delafraz, Santa Monica, CA.

Printed in the United States of America

Dedication

This book is dedicated to John Graves, my super man. Thank you for your endless support and immense wisdom and love. You're my rock and my voice of reason. I thank God for you every day!

I would also like to dedicate this book to Dr. Alicia Stanton, a truly beautiful woman - both inside and out. Although you are no longer with us, you will always be a mentor to me. Even during your final months you remained a joyful, positive light. Your insight and expertise will continue to inspire me. I thank you for your support, advice, and graciously taking precious time to write the 'Foreword' for this book. You will be missed, my colleague and shining star.

Disclaimer & Important Note to the Reader

This publication contains the opinions and ideas of its author. It is intended to provide helpful and informational material on the subject matter covered. This is not a medical reference book, and not meant to be a substitution for diagnosis, discussion or treatment by a medical physician or professional and not intended to treat, cure or prevent any disease. As the reader, you assume all risk and liability resulting from the use or misuse of all information provided herein including but not limited to supplements, recipes, health or beauty products, treatments, exercises or equipment noted within these pages.

If you have health concerns, take medications, have a medical, hormonal or skin condition, if planning to be or are pregnant, breast-feeding, or diagnosed bi-polar or depressed, consult your physician or health care provider before using the information herein. For those with allergies or who experience an irritation or adverse reaction to any product or beauty recipe or supplement noted herein, discontinue use, remove any product with soap and water and immediately consult a dermatologist or personal physician.

The information noted herein is without guarantee on the part of the author, publisher or distributor. Publisher, distributors, author, owners and/or representatives of hollywoodbeautysecrets.com, hollywoodbeautysecrets.net, beautylifechanger.com, louisagraves.com, and their heirs will not be held responsible for any liability, loss, injury, judgment, medical or legal costs, expenses, fees or payments in connection with the use or misuse of the information herein. The products and information noted throughout this book have not been evaluated or approved by the FDA, except the Led Red Light Therapy unit. Use the information at your own risk.

Contents

Foreword
by Alicia Stanton, MD

"Louisa Graves is a Beauty and Age-proofing Expert who fo-
cuses on science and the recommendations of the medical
community to reveal and, in some cases help create the most
effective choices available to us for the care of our face, hands,
feet, nails, hair and body. In addition, many of her beauty solutions are simple with common ingredients that are easy to find.
Louisa is a well known hands and body parts model in Hollywood and in order to stay on top of her game she has done
countless hours of research to find out what REALLY works to
enhance beauty and reduce the effects of aging. We are very fortunate that Louisa has chosen to share her proven research
with us! Louisa has also worked diligently to uncover a number
of wonderful products she offers at budget-friendly prices to the
public through her website. As a physician who specializes in
hormone balance and nutrition, I really appreciate the care she
has taken to focus on the beneficial effects of certain nutrients
for the hair, skin and nails. Most importantly, many products
she recommends do not contain any Bisphenol A or phthalates.
These toxins are found in many other hair and skin care products and are known to cause disruption in the balance of many
of our hormones.

I would feel very comfortable recommending Louisa's products
to my patients and I use many of them myself. I congratulate
Louisa on her many accomplishments and thank her for sharing her wisdom and beauty secrets with all of us!"

Alicia Stanton, MD

Fellow American College of Obstetrics and Gynecology
Diplomat of the Board of Anti-Aging Medicine
Advanced Fellow in Anti-Aging and Regenerative Medicine
International Speaker
Author of *The Complete Idiot's Guide to Hormone Weight Loss*

Introduction
Celebrity Body Parts Model-Turned-Beauty Expert

I'm often asked how I became a top beauty expert and author. It all began in Hollywood, during my career as a celebrity body parts model. What many don't know is that those close-up shots of hands and body parts as seen on TV are quite often mine! I've doubled my hands and body parts for 100's of Hollywood actresses and A-list stars in over 1000 commercials, movies and television shows. Some of those stars include *Jennifer Garner, Penelope Cruz, Kate Walsh, Gwyneth Paltrow, Courtney Thorne-Smith, Alyssa Milano, Debra Messing, Andie MacDowell, Cindy Crawford, Milla Jovovich, Heather Locklear, Kirstie Alley, and one of the Desperate Housewives - just to name a few!*

As you can imagine, keeping my skin in camera-ready shape was, and still continues to be, a part of my daily routine. Though I'm a busy beauty expert in the media, I still get calls from producers and directors to double my hands and parts. My secret? I use many of the products, beauty foods, safe supplements and stress-busting protocols noted within this book. So I guess you could say that I 'walk the talk.' Given the reactions I receive from women that I meet in person, I am pleased to say that my non-invasive tips are working. ☺

You'll discover a variety of age-proofing tips, beauty gadgets that *really* work, and weight loss and hormone-balancing devices that you can use in the privacy of your home. My tips are revolutionary and concise. The products noted are accessible and <u>affordable</u>. You will learn which toxic skin care and household products every woman (and family) should avoid *how to make your own healthy household products *how to rid your body of toxins and reduce stress *the best brain boosters, good mood foods and drug-free hormone-balancing tips that cost pennies *how to naturally increase energy *safe and effective supplements *how to repair and prevent wrinkles *how to achieve uninterrupted sleep *build bone density and firm muscles - just 10 minutes a day *firm sagging and thinning skin *ignite fat-burning *reduce enlarged pores and blemishes *prevent acne and fade pigmentation spots *rejuvenate hands *halt thinning hair *banish cracked heels, chapped lips, puffy eyes, cellulite and much more.

I also share hundreds of my favorite beauty recipes, age-proofing remedies and delicious meals and snacks made with natural ingredients throughout and at the back of this book. In addition, I have provided accessible resources where you can purchase ingredients, supplements and cutting-edge products in **Safe, Effective Face & Body Product Suggestions**. I even offer some of the harder-to-find products on my web site shop at discount prices. Please view my free beauty videos at www.Youtube.com/user/BeautyGuru/videos and sign up for my free monthly newsletter at www.HollywoodBeautySecrets.com. If you have an iPhone or iPad download my **Hollywood Beauty Secrets® app** noted on the back cover of this book.

I'm an Ingredients Sleuth

I've spent many years researching age-defying ingredients, supplements and formulations that are scientifically proven. Best of all - they don't cost an arm and a leg! Whether you're a new mom, a baby boomer or senior citizen, my tips can help you feel and look your best. Thousands of women who have used my beauty secrets, report that they feel more energized and empowered, look and feel more beautiful, confident, and ready to take on life's day to day challenges with a more uplifted attitude and much less stress! I am honored to share my tips and research with you. Enjoy! Louisa

NOTE: At the time of writing this book, I was not a paid spokesperson for any of the products noted in these pages. Please be sure to read the disclaimer before using the information herein.

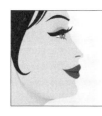

Age-Proofing Tip #1
Keep Good Thoughts

Our health and wellbeing is a result of our choices and actions. Each action we take begins with a thought.

Many physicians agree that positive thoughts can improve all aspects of our lives. Negative thinking darkens our daily paths and can manifest into fear, anxiety, stress, failure and other limitations. Over time, negative thinking becomes a *habit* that can hinder relationships, goals and our health. Did you know that being surrounding with argumentative, emotionally unstable, negative or dramatic individuals, can affect your mental wellbeing and weaken your immune system?

Several scientific studies have proven that we can re-program our *subconscious* minds to attract whatever we desire in life. By letting go of negative thoughts and personalities we can transform into more optimistic, successful and healthy individuals. Several spiritual and metaphysical books such as those written by Florence Shinn, Emmett Fox and Ernest Holmes have been sharing this 'new thought' movement since the early 1900s. Their writings have influenced millions of individuals worldwide, including many of today's spiritual and self-help doctors, speakers and authors.

How we think can transform our lives. Personal enhancement, peace, enlightenment, prosperity and much more can be achieved by adjusting our thoughts. Celebrate each day as an opportunity to start over, to make progress toward a goal and to make positive, life-altering choices. Positive thinking renews the mind and body. It is age-proofing!

"Everything's in the mind. That's where it all starts. Knowing what you want is the first step toward getting it." – Mae West

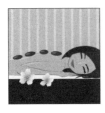

Age-Proofing Tip #2
Make Time for You

Life keeps us very busy. But due to our hectic schedules, many of us often neglect to take time for ourselves. Ongoing stress can affect our health, self-esteem and our disposition. It can trigger sadness, moodiness, and impatience. For many busy women, weight gain is usually the result of stress-related binge eating and if not addressed, can lead to feelings of hopelessness, anxiety and even depression.

Taking a daily 'time out' halts stress. It can improve our health, uplift our spirits, and build self-esteem and confidence. When we feel calm and happy, it shows on the outside and affects every aspect of our lives. Looking and feeling our best is vital to our mental and physical health. By making healthy choices including the foods we eat, the thoughts we think and incorporating time for ourselves - our health will not only improve, we will become more energized, positive and empowered. In addition, making time for you can prevent disease and weight gain.

Your Body is Your Temple

In order to be at your best, set aside time each day to nourish and strengthen your body and calm your thoughts. As you will read in **Age-Proofing Tip #4**, repeating a specific routine for just 14 days is habit forming. I urge you to dedicate 30 or 40 minutes a day to walk, stretch, do yoga or go to the gym. After just two weeks, you'll be hooked. If your schedule is tight or you're a stay-at-home mom, check out several effective at-home exercises noted in **Age-Proofing Tip #57.** If your budget allows, take yoga or pilates classes, or use a Body Vibration Plate. One 10-minute workout on a vibration plate is the equivalent of jogging five miles but without the stress on your knees and hips. Vibration therapy can help balance hormones, build bone density, reduce cellulite, rapidly tone muscles and more. Find out more benefits of Body Vibration Plates in **Age-Proofing Tip #58.**

Below are more tips on how you can gain more you time.

Ask Your Family for Help

It's a fact that the busiest women find it difficult to ask for help from others. Moms will do whatever it takes to provide for their children and spouses. Now what if the situation were reversed?

6

Would you ask your spouse/partner and children to help you with household chores? Do you think they would help if you asked? Of course they would! Ask and you shall receive! No need to be superwoman 24/7.

Useful phrases such as "would you please help me with this?" or "I could really use your help" - are very effective. These phrases allow them the opportunity to say no, though I think your loving approach will surely result in a yes.

Family Basics

It's important for all of us to gain some basic life skills - children included. Once your little ones reach the age of eight or so, set up a weekly 'family training' session. Be sure to get your spouse/partner involved too. Cleaning and organizing, mopping floors, doing dishes, and preparing healthy snacks and simple meals are skills everyone can master. In addition, you'll create the perfect opportunity for you and your spouse to open up a dialogue with your children. Casually ask about their friends and school activities. Ask their opinion about a topic. We all need to be heard. This is a great time to listen to your child's positive or negative thoughts. Remember- negative thoughts can become a habit. Help them kick the negativity habit by steering them in the healthier direction - becoming more positive and grateful individuals. After a few family training sessions your family will become even closer, more self-sufficient and positive, AND you'll free up some 'time for you.' See? Everyone benefits.
Below are more family training tips:

-Set up a weekly family cooking lesson. Prepare <u>three</u> healthy meals and snacks. If your spouse doesn't cook, this will be good training for him too. Within a month every member of your family will know how to prepare at least 12 nutritional meals;

-Younger children can set and clear the table or take the garbage out;

-Your spouse/partner can help with dishes, do laundry or drive the kids to soccer practice or music lessons, etc;

-Teens can vacuum their rooms and do their own laundry. Just show them how to sort colors, use the washer and dryer, and leave them be;

-Show your children how to organize and take care of their belongings. This instills responsibility and a sense of pride; and

-Create a 'Make Time for You' schedule with your spouse. This way you can both schedule some down time.

Be sure to acknowledge your family's help. Saying, "thank you" for even the smallest chore can yield big results. Acknowledgement is the key. Now instead of rushing home after work, once or twice a week, do something for you. Take a yoga class, get a massage, or take a walk around your neighborhood. Some nights, just come home and take an hour to unwind. Indulge in a relaxing bath or take a nap. You get the idea. Taking time to 'decompress' is essential for peak health. Most importantly, when you feel relaxed, home becomes a peaceful paradise for all.

"Time you enjoy wasting, was NOT wasted." – John Lennon

Mindful Children Become Thoughtful Adults

By teaching children the basics in cooking and cleaning or how to be more organized, they'll use these helpful life skills when they leave the 'nest' for college. They'll be self-sufficient, more mindful room mates, and perfectly capable of preparing nourishing meals for themselves. Now don't you feel better about family training?

FACT: New research reveals that husbands and children have adapted to becoming more self-sufficient around the home. A study published by Fortune Magazine noted, *"Of the 187 participants at Fortune's Most Powerful Women in Business summit last spring, 30 % had househusbands."*

A Model Husband

My husband can run circles around me, thanks in part to his mom. Thank you, Patty! By the time he moved out at age 18, he knew how to cook, do laundry, clean house, mow the lawn, paint, and much more. He's the king of multi-tasking - a likely reason for his success running restaurants and his own coffee shops.

Being a former stand-up comic, he keeps me laughing too. He is my business partner, takes care of our home, and he's an amazing cook too. Now that's what I call a *super* man. I've shared some of his recipes in **My Favorite Healthy Meal & Snack Recipes**. With his support and thoughtfulness I can take time for me. I've often said, "Johnnie, you need to write a book about how to be the best husband on earth." He just looks at me and says, "A happy wife is a happy husband."

Be grateful for your partner's / family's help around the house. By showing appreciation, for even the littlest deeds, don't be surprised to find a clean house and a nice meal waiting for you on a regular basis. Now go take some time for you! ☺

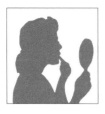

Age-Proofing Tip #3
Embrace Your Authenticity

When you look in the mirror, do you love who you see? Or do you wish you looked younger or were a dress size smaller?

Why are women so critical of themselves? Why do we compare ourselves to other women? Men don't do that! As a beauty expert I talk with many women on a daily basis and I often find myself reminding them that being beautiful is a *mind set*. Beauty is not defined by our weight or dress size. Many women will go to dangerous or costly extremes including countless cosmetic surgery procedures or starvation diets to pursue 'perfection'. Achieving perfection is unrealistic, unhealthy and unattainable. Looking and feeling our best IS attainable. It's time to stop wishing away our 40s, 50s or 60s. Instead, let's embrace and celebrate who we are and how we appear *now!* From this moment on- let's make a pact to be kind and gentle with ourselves.

Embracing your authenticity and loving yourself *now* creates an inner peacefulness and gentleness that manifests into true beauty, inside and out.

Switch Gears from Over-Critical

Beginning today, when you look in the mirror, focus on your feminine curves, your bright eyes, that gorgeous smile, or maybe your 'fashionista' sense! You don't have to go 'under the knife' or spend a fortune to look and feel your best. If you want to make some small changes - that's perfectly okay too. Sometimes one little change can make a world of difference.

Consider a new hairstyle, color, or make-over. Study hairstyles and makeup in fashion magazines. Then tear out the pages and book a consultation with your stylist and a professional makeup artist.

TIP: When you see a woman with a great haircut or color, ask where she gets her hair done! You'll not only uplift her day, you may have just found a new hair stylist!

If your goal is to get into better physical shape, turn to someone who looks fit. When I see a fabulous and fit-looking woman, I'll just walk up to her and say, "You look amazing! What's your secret?" I've picked up so many tips this way. If you're a stay-at-home mom and can't get to the gym, seek other moms in your neighborhood and start a walking group - strollers and all. If you have a job, ask a co-worker to walk with you during your lunch breaks. If your budget allows, seek the advice of a nutritionist or hire a trainer to create a workout routine and menu for you.

Now go out there, take positive steps toward your goal(s), and most importantly - embrace yourself along your path. Let your positive, beautiful journey unleash.

"At any age inner beauty radiates out through positive words and intentions. The more I focus on inner beauty, the more I attract beautiful expressions in my life. From this elevated awareness, I convey genuine peace and balance." – Daily Word

A Note about Beauty & Change from Dr. Robert Puff, Clinical Psychologist

For a moment, let's imagine our beauty is an open field. Beauty is a gift from God. It's something we can celebrate and be excited about. However, we may want to change and make some improvements - or we may not. Either one is fine. If we decide, *"Yes my hair is graying a bit. I think I'll color my hair to cover the gray"* it is okay; or we can say *"Yes, my hair is graying but I'm just going to accept it. I don't mind the graying"*- then that's okay too. But do you see the gentleness there? We're kind about our looks. We can change them but we can also love them and keep them the same. We can be excited about change or excited about aging naturally. Both can be fine but if we don't accept what we have, even after the improvements, we are going to be unhappy. I think that's where we need to be careful about media and advertisements. They play on our insecurities. Health is about accepting what is and ultimately loving what is.

Beauty is something that we can change, we can improve upon, and we can accept. But to be happy, to have a good life, we need to love what we have and/or love the improvements we make with what we have. If every time we look in the mirror we are self-critical, we attack ourselves and say things like, "That's ugly. That's unattractive. Those wrinkles are just disgusting" then we're going to suffer. Instead, say "Hey, that's a beautiful person there. I love that person and I'm going to make some changes and make that person FEEL even more beautiful!"

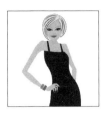

Age-Proofing Tip #4
Take Pride in Your Appearance

Medical experts agree that taking care of our appearance is emotionally uplifting. One of the first lessons taught to those seeking counseling for depression is to follow a daily grooming regimen. Psychological studies have proven that the simple act of applying makeup, washing our hair and changing into nice clothes, can transform our mental wellbeing and our outlook on life. Repetition is <u>the</u> key. After following a daily grooming regimen for just <u>two weeks</u>, it becomes an instinctively positive action that helps reverse depression. The same goes for exercise. After two weeks of daily exercise you'll be 'in the groove.'

In addition, how we present ourselves affects how others perceive us. **Below are some facts you'll find eye-opening.**

-A popular job website article noted that… "A well-groomed person is 60% more likely to get a job, over a more qualified candidate that appears disheveled or un-groomed."

-Another study noted that we perceive a well-groomed, well-dressed person to be more attractive, honest and trustworthy.

-An article in *The Economist* noted that… "Attractive people are judged to be more intelligent; they earn more, and are more likely to marry."

-Several studies have proven that taking pride in our appearance uplifts our mood, increases confidence and leads to more success in life.

Putting it to the Test

I decided to test the grooming theory. I styled my hair, put on some makeup, a stylish dress and heels, and headed out the door to a local grocery store. I must admit, I felt really good. As I walked down the store aisles with a smile on my face and a spring in my step, every employee I passed smiled back at me AND asked if I needed any help. In addition, several customers engaged in conversations with me. One gal asked how I stayed in shape, one man complimented my shoes - and my legs. Hee hee. Another woman stopped and asked where I bought my dress. We spoke at length. It turned out that we both had a mutual admiration for 'wrap' dresses. She even told me about a website that offered them on sale. I also got help out to my car. The experience kept me smiling for the rest of the day.

"Happiness and self-confidence are true measures of attractiveness." – Mertz/Harris Survey

A few days later I walked into the same store, but this time I sported sweats, running shoes, no makeup and my hair was tied in a messy pony tail. The employees were the same ones that noticed me just days before. But this time, as I walked up and down the aisles (sans smile), not one person acknowledged me. Wow - that was an eye-opener!

Putting your best self 'out there' is empowering and can open the door to endless possibilities.

LOUISA GRAVES

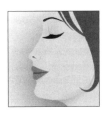

Age-Proofing Tip #5
My Daily Feel Good Ritual

I love to read metaphysical books. They are empowering. Since incorporating the ideas of these spiritual writers, my life has changed. I feel more calm and enriched. I have let go of worry or putting pressure on myself, and I have reduced stress in my life. I wake up feeling excited and confident about what each day will bring! Most importantly, I have learned that the key to happiness, success, and peak health is to let go of fear or doubt, to love what I do, get plenty of rest, be spontaneous and enjoy life in the moment.

In addition, I like to pray each morning and evening, nourish my body with healthy foods, and make time to pamper myself. I now work less and play more. And since doing so, I have achieved <u>more</u> success and happiness *and* I feel and look better!

Each day, life keeps us busy with challenges and decisions. If feeling unhappy or fearful in a situation such as a job, relationship, or life in general, we each have the tools to improve many, if not all, of these circumstances. However, in some special cases, if feeling hopeless, sad, or unable to move past a trauma that has left you in a 'trapped' or anxious state, I urge you to seek professional counseling as soon as possible. These feelings may be a sign of hormone imbalance or depression and are more common that you would think. Please do not hesitate to seek help.

We are each worthy of divine happiness, health and success.

Create Your Heaven on Earth

For me, performing a calming ritual each morning and evening sets the tone for overcoming just about every challenge, including running my own business. It has helped keep my thoughts positive, improving every aspect of my life. Call it what you will - a mantra, or subconscious re-programming. I call it my daily feel good ritual. After performing my ritual, I can't wait to start my day to see what great experiences will unfold. And each day, they do! My thoughts and actions have helped me create a life-changing path - I'm creating my 'heaven' on earth.

14

When to do my Daily Feel Good Ritual

The best time to perform this ritual is at night - just before falling asleep, and again in the morning - just before rising from bed. This is when the *subconscious* mind is open to accepting good, positive thoughts. The subconscious mind is like a sponge. You can re-program and absorb new thoughts and feelings by repeating your desires and prayers every day. Within weeks, or even just days, your life can begin to transform. The smallest thought can trigger a big change. You will soon notice that what you focus on - is what you will attract. So why not focus on good things and what you do want! It's very exciting and uplifting to witness wonderful events manifesting each day.

Below, I've noted some examples of what you might repeat to yourself each morning and evening:

If you're going to a job interview or desire an increase in pay, repeat…*"I will be given my ultimate dream job and salary"* or *"I will get this job (or raise)"* or *"I am drawing success and prosperity toward me."*

If you're feeling under the weather, repeat something like…*"I am healing my body"* or *"I am drawing perfect health toward me."*

If feeling insecure, repeat …*"I reclaim my inner power"* or *"I am strong and intelligent and have a lot to offer."*

If unable to forgive or holding onto anger, or resentment repeat…*"I am letting go of pain and anger and I forgive _____ (their name)"* or *"I claim my new path to happiness."*

If your weight loss plan is not providing the results you desire, repeat…*"I am taking positive steps to manage my weight"* or *"I am gentle with myself on my weight loss journey."*

If you want to meet Mr. Right, repeat…*"I am attracting THE man/partner who will love and adore me, and I him."*

Or my favorites…*"I am open to changes and opportunities today"* or *"I will see good in others and keep positive thoughts today."*

*Another daily ritual is writing down your thoughts in a journal. Not sure what to write? List all the things in life that you are grateful for each day, such as your health, a loving family, access to healthy foods, your friends, a good salary and career you enjoy. You get the idea. Journaling can help calm your thoughts.

*Don't dwell on the past. Life's precious moments are NOW.

"The brightest future will always be based on a forgotten past: you cannot go forward until you let go of your past failures and heartaches." – Anonymous

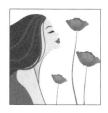

Age-Proofing Tip #6
Manage Stress for Better Health,
Rejuvenation & Weight Loss

"Once thoughts are in order, the world is your oyster!"

Our bodies respond to our thoughts and feelings. When we're feeling down our bodies become tired and sometimes even sick. When we feel positive, our bodies are healthier; we become uplifted, more energized and enthusiastic about life. If you have a hectic lifestyle or occupation, I urge you to read the following life-changing tips that can help you feel less stressed, more energized and rejuvenated.

The Stress, Weight Gain & Brain Fog Connection

Living in a constant state of stress not only rapidly ages us; it affects our health and hormones, impairs memory, and causes weight gain. Continuous stress causes the body to naturally release a hormone called cortisol. As stress prolongs we experience brain fog, irritability and sadness as well as additional inches of fat on the waist, hips and thighs. This can be devastating for many women.

Our stress hormone cortisol, provides energy. But when produced in excess, cortisol blocks the thyroid hormone which regulates how quickly we burn calories. This hinders weight loss, increases belly fat, water retention <u>and</u> cravings for high-carbohydrate foods such as sweets and starchy foods. These high glycemic and caloric comfort foods stimulate our endorphins (feel-good transmitters) in the brain, providing a <u>temporary</u> high that calms us for a short time. However, high-carb foods enter the blood stream quickly and cause blood sugar spikes that stimulate the production of insulin. When insulin levels rise, the body's ability to burn fat <u>slows</u> down. As this cycle continues, the pancreas eventually stops producing the correct supply of insulin the body requires, which can lead to diabetes. In addition, sugar and high-carbohydrate foods cause inflammation and aged-looking skin, low energy, sore joints and even some diseases. **NOTE:** If you are prone to acne, spikes in blood sugar trigger an increase in testosterone production which causes more oil production and results in acne and blemish-breakouts. Read more about the importance of consuming low to medium GI (glycemic index) foods in **Age-Proofing Tip #54.**

Ongoing Stress & Adrenal Exhaustion

Incorporating a healthy diet and avoiding high-carb comfort foods can enhance your health and wellbeing. However, if stressed-out for long periods of time (weeks to months), the constant output of cortisol will sabotage those good dietary habits resulting in added inches of fat to the waist and hips. Continued stress exhausts the adrenal system leading to a variety of health concerns such as depression, fatigue, thyroid issues, brain fog, panic attacks, irritability, low libido, restlessness, weight gain and more. Please visit your doctor if experiencing these symptoms. Author, Dr. Alicia Stanton, outlines some excellent tips for addressing adrenal exhaustion in her book, *"The Complete Idiots' GUIDE TO: Hormone Weight Loss,"* available at bookstores.

Reading Emails Increases Stress & Our Waistlines

Did you know that reading emails increases stress? One study revealed that the anticipation of what's in an email causes cortisol production to rise. In addition, those annoying unsolicited emailed advertisements prey on our fears, increasing anxiety even further.

Everywhere we look someone is texting, tweeting, emailing or phoning someone else. I've witnessed 'texters' causing traffic accidents and bumping into others. One gal even tripped and fell into a mall fountain while texting and walking! Even worse, many individuals talk on their phones while eating, mindlessly gulping down their food. Others text while on a coffee break. Isn't a coffee 'break' our time to relax and breathe - to get away from the phones, computers, tweets and emails? These electronic gadgets have definitely got an unhealthy hold on us!

Why can't we sit quietly, relax and just be? Do we fear that we'll miss out on something big? Honestly, whatever we may be anticipating - *will* happen when the time is *right* - when God and the universe make it happen.

Electronic Devices and the Weight Gain Connection

The reality is, to do our jobs many of us must rely on phones, computers and other electronic devices. But the sad truth is that when we're 'on' for countless hours a day, our bodies spew out cortisol. This can drain the adrenal system, cause anxiety, sleeplessness, over eating, and cravings for junk food which affects our wellbeing and increases our waistlines. Given the ever increasing rise in obesity rates I often wonder if using electronic devices are another cause of this sky-rocketing phenomenon. Read the alarming obesity statistic below. It's something to think about. Who doesn't have a cell phone or computer?

FACT: *In the USA, adult obesity rates increased in 16 states during the past year and none of the 50 states showed any decline in their rates of obesity.*

If your job requires communicating via email or phone, take two moments each hour of the day to do my **'Waist' Management De-stressing Ritual,** noted in **Age-Proofing Tip #7**. It's a quick and effective way to switch off cortisol and to re-set your self back to calm mode. I also recommend that if you have a high-stress schedule to begin your day with meditation or prayer. Try my daily feel good ritual noted in **Age-Proofing Tip #5.** In addition, set boundaries while away from work. Turn your cell phone off during lunch. Take a quiet 10-15 minute walk by yourself. Walking is a scientifically proven stress buster as noted in **Age-Proofing Tip #8.**

Consider turning your computer and phones off after 7:00 p.m. Time away from work is *your time.* Calm your mind, nourish your body and just be. This will result in a more focused, healthier and rejuvenated YOU.

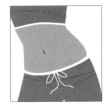

Age-Proofing Tip #7
'Waist' Management De-stressing Ritual

During days when you feel tension rising, a great way to instantly halt this is by performing my two-minute de-stressing ritual. You can do this while sitting at your desk or work station. Within seconds you'll feel immediate calm *and* switch off cortisol production! Perform my two minute ritual every hour of your work day to combat ongoing stress. If you work eight hours, this will take just 16 minutes a day. That's a small amount of time to ensure good mental and physical health and wellbeing. You can also do this on a subway ride to or from work, or while sitting in a parked car. **Here's what to do:**

While sitting, close your eyes and drop your shoulders down and back slightly. Then count to five, inhale slowly through your nose, breathing into your stomach - not your chest. Then, count to five again as you breathe out slowly through your nose. Be sure to keep your shoulders down as you breathe. TIP: Counting to five helps you focus <u>away</u> from stressful thoughts. After just <u>two minutes</u> you will feel the tension leaving your body. Another bonus of this exercise is that it can help those challenged with constipation. Breathing into the belly relaxes the intestines.

I enjoy my career very much. However, I sometimes receive 50-100 emails a day. Along with the usual day to day operations of running a business, doing consultations, interviews, writing articles, and appearing on TV shows, I am well aware that though I love what I do, my busy schedule can cause underlying stress! To address this, I have conditioned myself to walk away from my computer every hour. I make a cup of tea or drink a glass of water and do a few stretches. I also incorporate my **De-stressing Ritual**.

In addition, each day I make sure to schedule some 'time for me.' Four days a week I will either take a walk or ride my bike. On days that I don't take a walk, I use my ***Body Vibration Plate*** for 20 minutes. It helps me sleep better and is a quick way to increase muscle tone and manage my weight. One evening a week I lay in my ***FIR infrared sauna blanket*** for relaxation, detoxifying my body, to enhance weight loss and clear skin. This is most helpful for all women, especially those with hormonal imbalances such as after child birth, during menopause or when feeling under the weather. It can help prevent sore muscles after a workout and halts the beginning signs of a cold or flu. Many hormone health doctors recommend FIR infrared sauna treatments to help eliminate toxins, calm the body and mind. Read more about Body Vibration Plates in **Age-Proofing Tip #58** and **FIR infrared sauna blankets in Age-Proofing Tip #59.**

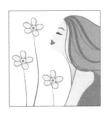

Age-Proofing Tip #8
Walking – the Scientifically Proven Stress-Buster

Another easy and effective way to halt stress is by taking a walk. It stimulates the endorphins, uplifts our mood and halts cortisol production. Walking is do-able and recommended for everyone - especially for those with hectic schedules, hormonal imbalances, adrenal exhaustion, and emotional or weight issues.

Whenever feeling tense, simply walk quietly for 20-40 minutes. You don't have to walk briskly or go to a gym. Walk anywhere, anytime. Get in touch with the earth, enjoy the flowers and trees, pray or meditate and *breathe.* You'll soon discover that walking is a calming, transforming experience. Keep a pair of walking shoes at work. Find top brands at discount department stores such as TJ Maxx® and Nordstrom Rack®.

Clinical psychologist, author and international speaker, Dr. Robert Puff, suggests walking in silence to 'unclutter our thoughts.' His training has helped many Fortune 500 executives improve their careers and life challenges. Quiet walking creates an environment which has been proven to calm the mind and in some cases stimulates ideas and thoughts that can solve concerns. Einstein took quiet walks to help solve mathematical equations. Walking in silence has helped me resolve daily challenges and is a perfect time to pray or meditate. Get in touch with your divine spirit - your inner self. Find Dr. Puff's DVDs and books at **TheHolisticSuccessShow.com**.

International walking guru, Manuela Stoerzer Vogt, has worked with many individuals challenged with severe burn-out, shock, nervous breakdown, depression and drug addiction. Her clients range from high powered executives, fatigued mothers and baby boomers, to patients in detox centers and mental health clinics. In all such cases, Manuela reveals that the physical experience of walking has been proven to overcome a number of traumatizing mental challenges. Walking helps her clients achieve positive mental thoughts that steer them away from stressful or negative mindsets, resulting in more joy and increased energy. Whether leading groups or taking clients out individually, Manuela walks in peaceful places such as hiking trails and on beaches, which provides a more calming, spiritual environment. Within a short period of time her clients incorporate walking regularly. The other benefits of walking include improved immune system, weight loss, reduced blood pressure and total body conditioning. Find out more at **Walkingguru.org.**

If weather won't allow for a walk outdoors, you have asthma, fibromyalgia or are a busy mom with little ones, incorporate breathing exercises such as yoga and stretching. Another cost-effective option is investing in a ***Body Vibration Plate.*** Read more about the health benefits of this life-changing device noted in **Age-Proofing Tip #58.** It is very affordable and can be done in the privacy of your home or office. I predict that within five years every household will have a Body Vibration Plate.

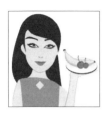

Age-Proofing Tip #9
Brain Boosters & Good Mood Foods

NOTE: check with your health care professional before taking suggested supplements.

Whether a stay-at-home mom, homemaker, or a career woman on the go, we are all super women! We make decisions, solve daily challenges, pay bills, and run our households, to name just a few responsibilities. The pressures of day to day life can be overwhelming and can cause irritability and even sadness. On top of all that, if you're a mother, you have even more on your plate. Working moms are the ultimate superwomen! I've often wondered how my mom managed to raise and care for five children by age 33 while working at the same time.

Address stress, nourish your body and uplift your spirits with good mood foods, safe supplements and soothing beverages as noted below.

Tryptophan is an essential amino acid that is found in many foods. It can enhance and calm our mood. It helps raise our serotonin levels, regulates anxiety, stress, insomnia, moodiness and even depression. Tryptophan can be taken as a time-released supplement and is also found in many healthy foods such as turkey, tofu, shrimp, chicken, tuna, cod, salmon, soybeans, asparagus, green beans and others noted below.

Pumpkin seeds contain stress-busting B vitamins, and plant-based omega 6s, which are beneficial for calming the nerves, and help with weight loss. They are high in protein and contain mood-uplifting ***tryptophan.* Enjoy pumpkin seeds as a snack when feeling stressed at work or as a pre-workout treat.

Walnuts are considered the ultimate nut for health, stress, mood and rejuvenation. They contain more omega 3 fatty acids than salmon, as well as protein, vitamin B, polyphenols and alpha lineolenic acid. These wonderful properties can calm muscles and nourish the adrenals. In addition, they help boost brain power and uplift mood. Walnuts make an excellent age-defying snack for calming and de-stressing or when experiencing brain fog or feeling 'blue.'

Brazil nuts are rich in selenium. Many studies conclude that low levels of selenium can cause depression. Eating one to two brazil nuts a day can uplift mood, reduce anxiety and even help keep arteries clear for peak heart health. Other foods rich in selenium include tuna and turkey.

Bananas are loaded with potassium to help maintain blood pressure and vitamin B6 to help calm stress. Eating a banana increases our serotonin levels - the feel good boosters in the brain. *Archives of Internal Medicine* notes that bananas can help prevent heart disease and contain properties that eliminate bacteria that cause ulcers. Bananas contain a natural sugar called frucooligo-saccharides (FOS) which is 50% less sweet than regular sugar, and unlike other sweeteners, is absorbed by the flora in the large intestine for nourishment and increased energy.

Besides being high in antioxidants and fiber, **pears** contain potassium which calms anxiety and lowers blood pressure. Recent research also reveals that compounds in white fruits such as pears and veggies such as cauliflower can help prevent strokes.

Cherries contain melatonin which calms and rejuvenates us, improves our memory, concentration, provides a more restful sleep and can even reduce muscle pain. According to a *University of Michigan* study, tart cherry juice can lower cholesterol, blood sugar levels and decreases fat storage in the liver which can aid weight loss.

Coconut Oil can do wonders for those challenged with brain fog or poor memory. Recent astounding studies reveal that consuming 1 tsp. of coconut oil per day along with a low carbohydrate diet, increases brain power and can help reverse the signs of dementia and Alzheimer's. Here's how: low carbohydrate diets increase ketone production which occurs when the body breaks down stored fat. Ketones have been scientifically proven to reduce brain plaque, increase blood flow, energy and brain power. Here's the best part - coconut oil is rich in medium-chain triglycerides (MCT). Eating coconut oil triggers the body to produce even higher amounts of ketones which is proving helpful to those with Parkinson's, MS, and Alzheimer's. For improved concentration and memory, start with 1 tsp. of raw organic food grade coconut oil each day at breakfast time. Cook with coconut oil too.

Blueberries offer several powerful antioxidants that are age-defying and help fight free radical damage in the brain, improving memory and brain power. A *Harvard study* revealed that consuming one cup of blueberries per day can help protect the brain's neurons to reduce inflammation associated with aging and dementia. Blueberries are low-glycemic and low in calories and their dark purple color is packed with flavonoids that are rich in beta-carotene, vitamin A, and fiber. Did you know that blueberries contain four times the antioxidant power of vitamin C? Their anti-inflammatory benefits make blueberries one of the ultimate age-defying fruits.

Quinoa is a gluten-free, tasty alternative to rice that contains mood uplifting *tryptophan*** and is very satisfying. It is low in carbs and low-glycemic so it enters the system slowly, providing a feeling of fullness, without the guilt or blood sugar spikes. Quinoa is very high in protein. Read more about it in **Age-Proofing Tip #53 - Super Foods.**

Flaxseeds are high in omega-3 fatty acids. Flaxseeds and oil help balance hormones, reduce inflammation, provide cardio-vascular health, uplift mood, ignite fat burning, promote regularity and prevent blood sugar spikes. The beauty of this fat is that it also slows the aging process, and keeps skin hydrated and more youthful looking. Take flaxseed oil supplements twice daily with breakfast and lunch or grind up flax seeds and sprinkle them onto salads, oatmeal, yogurt, or add them to multi-grain pancake or bran muffin recipes. See my healthy low-glycemic, wheat-free pancakes in **My Favorite Healthy Meal & Snack Recipes.**

Lentils are high in *tryptophan*** plus fiber and minerals. They are fat-free and can help reduce cholesterol. Read more health benefits about lentils in **Age-Proofing Tip #53 - Super Foods**.

Spinach is a low-calorie, yet highly nutritious vegetable that is loaded with folic acid, iron, lutein manganese, *tryptophan***, vitamins A and K. These properties support eye and bone health and prevent oxidative inflammation which enhances brain power, and slows aging. New studies also suggest that the anti-oxidants in spinach may reduce the development breast and ovarian cancer as well as memory loss.

Eggs are high in protein and choline for muscle tone and nervous system function. Eggs also help boost memory and concentration.

Rescue Remedy® (Original Flower formulation) is a gentle and safe tonic derived from wild plants and herbs. When taken orally, it can help overcome daily feelings of anxiety, irritability or stress. It's available in spray, drops, or pastilles to help provide a soothing and calming effect for emotional support. Use it before doing a presentation or a public speaking event. When feeling under the weather, a few drops of Rescue Remedy® can uplift mood. Studies have proven that an uplifted mood helps us recover from physical illness more quickly. Developed by Dr. Robert Bach over 80 years ago, Rescue Remedy® was formulated as an effective medication alternative to address emotional wellbeing. Find it at your local health food store.

Ginkgo Biloba is a powerful antioxidant-rich herb that protects the neurons in the brain and improves brain power. It's been used in Eastern medicine for many decades to protect the brain from free radicals. Other bonuses of ginkgo biloba include increased fat burning and energy, improved eye sight and hearing, and is known to help prevent senility and Alzheimer's. To increase cognitive function, combining **cayenne** with **ginkgo biloba** is the ultimate brain booster. This dynamic duo stimulates healthy circulation in the brain, and reduces foggy memory by increasing the blood flow which clears plaque buildup and toxins that can settle in the brain. Renowned formulator, Dr. Schulze of American Botanical Pharmacy® in Marina del Rey, CA combines ginkgo biloba and cayenne in a formulation called **Brain**. It's available online at herbdoc.com.

Hibiscus Tea can help calm mood. One study noted that drinking two to three cups of hibiscus tea daily can reduce blood pressure and hypertension. Hibiscus tea, whether hot or iced, can even help cool down hot flashes. Another refreshing stress-busting tea alternative is combining hibiscus with pomegranate tea. **Here's what you do:**

Boil one cup of water and steep 2 hibiscus and 2 pomegranate tea bags for 15 minutes. Then pour the tea (with the tea bags) into a large glass carafe of water and let cool in the refrigerator. Pour some of this refreshing tea into a BPA-free water bottle and take it with you to work. Delicious! Find both teas at most health food stores.

Chamomile tea is a perfect non-caffeinated nightly beverage. It helps digestion and relieves anxiety by providing a calming effect.

Valerian Root Tea is an excellent pre-bedtime calming tea choice. Find it at your local health food store.

Kava can be taken as an herbal supplement or as tea to help calm the mind and body. It's an effective muscle relaxant and pain reducer and can enhance memory and mood. When taken in moderation it will not induce sleep during the day, though in higher amounts, can provide a better sleep.

St. John's Wort tea is known to help remedy mood swings or mild to moderate depression. You should start to feel relief after about one month of use. Find St. John's Wort tea bags at a local health food store. **NOTE:** Do not use St. John's Wort before surgery or if you're taking prescription anti-depressants.

Both sandalwood and lavender essential oils are aromatic, homeopathic oils that can help calm both the nervous system and mind. Spray either oil onto sheets to induce sleep or keep a little vial of either oil in your purse for emergencies. When stressed, or feeling a headache coming on, simply uncap either vial and take in the calming natural scents. Rubbing a little lavender on the temples can help reduce headaches too.

Vitamin D prevents depression, uplifts your mood and offers many more health benefits. It breaks down fat in the liver and reduces food cravings to help with weight loss goals, reduces the risk of breast and colon cancer by 30-50%, reduces eczema and psoriasis, throbbing or migraine headaches, rheumatoid arthritis, aids the immune system and increases energy. New studies reveal that it may even prevent a heart attack. Read about more benefits of vitamin D in **Age-Proofing Tip #51.**

Vitamin B5 (pantothenic acid) is an excellent supplement for mood uplifting and energy. It's highly recommended during all stages of menopause, and helps support the adrenal glands which produce and secrete cortisol, estrogen, adrenaline, and testosterone hormones. Vitamin B5 helps convert carbohydrates (sugars, starches) and fats into energy. It's even used by athletes for energy. Take vitamin B5 with breakfast or lunch along with your other vitamins. Find B5 in foods such as eggs, avocados, yogurt, corn, broccoli, sweet potatoes, bananas, and nuts. **NOTE:** Consuming sugar-laden foods decreases B vitamins. Avoid sugar when stressed.

Vitamin B6 can be taken at bedtime to help reduce cortisol levels and improve sleep patterns, ensuring uninterrupted rest. When taken daily B6 helps relieve mental fatigue, increases energy, reduces mood swings, keeps the immune system healthy, and improves memory. Find B6 in several foods such as bell peppers, spinach and summer squash. **NOTE:** Vitamin B6 is the only B vitamin recommended at bedtime.

CoQ10 can help those who feel tired or out of energy. CoQ10 is a powerful antioxidant that strengthens the muscles of the heart and is known to help those challenged with migraine headaches and Parkinson's disease. CoQ10 is also recommended for women taking the pill for birth control and those who wish to lose weight. Read more about CoQ10 in **My Favorite Supplements for Women.**

Rhodiola Extract has been used in Europe for centuries as a natural health-booster and to reduce fatigue or depression. It is very useful to those who live stressful, hectic lifestyles or when feeling 'blue'. Rhodiola enhances memory function, increases serotonin levels and emotional energy, reduces anxiety, and supports the adrenal system. It even increases memory power and concentration which is why many students and medical interns take this supplement. One study noted that students achieved higher test scores when taking rhodiola. Medical professionals take rhodiola to increase energy and mental performance and athletes use it for both stamina and physical fitness. Rhodiola is derived from a nutrient-packed plant.

Ashwagandha Root is an herbal supplement that reduces cortisol associated with stress and anxiety. It is beneficial for those challenged with high stress, weight issues, underactive thyroid, insomnia, low energy or brain fog.

5-HPT signals messages through the nervous system promoting a positive, uplifted mood throughout the day, and a calmer, rested feeling at night. It's a natural 'feel-good' neurotransmitter that is derived from plants. It is non-addictive, unlike prescription drugs. Some brands of 5-HTP are combined with stress-busting B-Vitamins. Another bonus of 5-HTP is it helps curb appetite and when taken at night, ensures a restful sleep. Read more about it in **Age-Proofing Tip #16 - Importance of Rejuvenating Sleep.**

Melatonin is a sleep hormone that the body naturally produces. It can improve the memory, helps lower blood pressure and is rejuvenating. Melatonin is a powerful antioxidant and anti-depressant supplement that regulates the immune system. It is recommended for those under stress or experiencing high cortisol production, brain fog or weight gain. It even boosts our brain power. Taking melatonin is safe and does not disrupt the body's natural production of melatonin though it can react with some medications, such as monoamine oxidize inhibitors (MOI's). **NOTE:** Do not take this supplement during the day as it causes drowsiness. Read more benefits of melatonin in **Age-Proofing Tip #16 - Importance of Rejuvenating Sleep.**

Gaba contains natural, safe, rejuvenating properties, increases concentration and can help reduce stress and anxiety. It can help to naturally relax the body and helps increase HGH (human growth hormone) production which substantially decreases once we hit age 40.

Magnesium is a diverse mineral with myriad benefits. Those who are challenged with anxiety, moodiness, sleeplessness, or depression can benefit from magnesium. Magnesium calms pain associated with fibromyalgia, migraine headaches, muscle and joint pain, and chronic fatigue. If challenged with constipation, magnesium can help loosen bowels. It even relieves water retention and protects bones, nerves and muscles. Find magnesium in dairy products and foods including figs, pumpkin seeds, spinach, swiss chard, soy and black beans. **NOTE:** If taking bone, thyroid or antibiotics, check with your physician for the best time to take magnesium. Read many more benefits of magnesium in **Age-Proofing Tip #16 - Importance of Rejuvenating Sleep.**

Sam-e (S-Adenosylmethionine), an amino acid, is a highly effective mood booster that can help with sadness, anger, moodiness or depression. Sam-e offers many other benefits with no known side effects. It supports joint health, brain function, and healthy connective tissue, cleanses the liver and can help slow the aging process by protecting DNA. For full potency make certain Sam-e is enteric coated and in a blister pack, not in a bottle. Take it on an empty stomach.

NOTE: Sam-e is not recommended for those challenged with manic depression (bi-polar) or currently taking anti-depressants. Ask your doctor about Sam-e.

For those challenged with adrenal exhaustion Michaelshealth.com offers an adrenal energy support supplement that combines ashwagandha root, pantothenic acid, Vitamin C and rhodiola extract.

NOTE: As noted in the disclaimer, check with your doctor before taking the supplements noted within these pages.

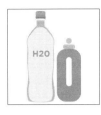

Age-Proofing Tip #10
Avoid BPA for Hormonal Health

BPA is a synthetic estrogen that disrupts the endocrine system, causing several health issues as noted below. Many household plastics including water and baby bottles, cellophane wrap, food storage containers and almost all food cans are manufactured with BPA (bisphenol A) resins. These resins can leach into our drinking water, beverages and foods. When BPA-formulated plastic containers are exposed to heat such as microwaving or sun exposure, the resins leach into the contents of those containers. Consuming BPA causes many hormonal imbalances. It can trigger early puberty and affect those going through stages of menopause or pregnancy. In addition, BPA has been linked to diabetes, weight gain and cancer.

Choose BPA-free food storage containers and cellophane wrap, and buy frozen vegetables or choose canned foods that note BPA-free packaging. Do not leave plastic water or baby bottles in the car exposed to sun or heat and never purchase bottled water that is stored outside of grocery stores exposed to sun. Many California supermarkets do this. I do my part and let the store managers know that exposing plastic water bottles to sun is not a safe practice.

How to Identify Safe Plastics

There are now many BPA-free plastic food storage containers and water bottles available to us. To be sure your plastic storage containers are BPA-free, locate the triangular symbol on the bottom of each container where you'll see a number noted. It is safe to store and heat foods in those marked number 2, 4 & 5. They are BPA-free. Avoid plastic bottles and containers marked 1, 3, 6, & 7 on the bottom. If no number is found, use the container to store non-food items such as paper clips, crayons, or hair accessories just to be safe.

Another option is to store and heat foods in glass dishware. And if re-heating foods in a microwave oven, use waxed paper or BPA-free cellophane wrap to cover dishware. Below is a partial list of food storage containers and plastic products that were tested and believed to contain no BPA. They are available in many grocery stores nationwide.

Gladware® Containers with Interlocking Lids *Glad® Simply Cooking Microwave Steaming Bags *Glad® Freezer Storage

Bags *Glad® Cling Wrap/Clear Plastic Wrap *Saran® Premium wrap *Saran® Cling Plus/Clear Plastic Wrap *Reynolds® Clear Seal-Tight Plastic Wrap *Ziploc® Brand Zip 'n' Steam Microwave and Steam Cooking Bags *Ziploc® Brand Containers with Snap 'N Seal Lids *Ziploc® Brand Storage Bags & Freezer Bags with Double Zipper.

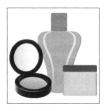

Age-Proofing Tip #11
Avoid Parabens

Parabens are added to thousands of grooming products including face creams and body lotions, sunscreens, deodorants, makeup, hair and bath products - just to name a few. They preserve the shelf life of products by preventing bacterial growth.

Many studies reveal that, when used in excess, parabens have been proven to affect our hormones and health. *Critical Reviews in Toxicology* notes that "parabens disrupt the human endocrine system and accumulate in our systems causing hormonal confusion." Also excessive use may lead to metabolic or neurological disorders. Dr. Alicia Stanton, author of, *"The Idiot's Guide to Hormone Weight Loss"* cautions women to avoid products containing parabens especially those who are pregnant, or going through hormonal changes.

Protect Mother Nature

Each day millions of Americans shower off products that contain parabens. These synthetic properties float down our drains and into the water system affecting Mother Earth too!

A study on wisegeek.com notes, "while parabens certainly do have estrogenic qualities, they are probably safe in *very small* amounts. Typically the concentration of parabens in cosmetics such as face creams and sun screens is very low, often less than 1%." So the good news is, when used *in moderation*, parabens are considered safe. However, startling statistics reveal that women on average use approximately 12 grooming products per day and over 90% of girls aged 14 begin using makeup, hair and body products.

Our skin is the largest body organ and it absorbs whatever we apply. The average-sized adult body is wrapped in approximately 20 square feet of skin! To reduce exposure, products that are used on the larger areas of the body, should be paraben free. They include sunscreen, deodorant, bath, body and hair products.

How to Detect Parabens in Products

When purchasing face, body and hair care products, read labels. Parabens are listed with these prefixes: Ethyl, Iso, Methyl, Propyl, or Butyl, and end with paraben. Drug stores now offer more paraben-free and organic products and I think this trend will continue as we voice our concerns.

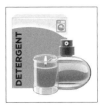

Age-Proofing Tip #12
Avoid Phthalates (Synthetic Fragrance)

Phthalates are added as fragrances to many commonly used products including face and body lotion, sunscreen, hairspray, shampoo, conditioner, makeup, soap, body wash, perfume, cologne, nail polish, candles, laundry detergent and household cleaners. One report noted that some deodorants, shampoos, aftershave and antibacterial soaps contain over 200 different synthetic chemicals. The *FDA* estimates that over 65% of cosmetics contain toxic ingredients. Research from *EWG.org* and the *Campaign for Safe Cosmetics* found an average of 14 to 17 chemicals in name brand fragrance products - yet none of these ingredients are listed on their labels! If you wear cologne or perfume, consider switching to natural, phthalate-free botanical essential oils available at all health food stores. I like **Oriental Musk** essential oil by **Kuumba Made®** and recommend **Amber and Sandalwood** for men.

More Startling Skin and Body Care Facts

-About a third of personal care products sold in the United States contain one or more ingredient with some evidence of being carcinogenic.

-With more than $45 billion in annual sales the United States is by far the world's largest market for cosmetics and toiletries.

-Women typically use 12 personal care products daily, twice as many as men.

-An estimated 90% of girls age 14 and older regularly use cosmetics.

Sources: Datamonitor, Environmental Working Group, Euromonitor International, The Economist, The American Medical Association, Kline & Co., Natural Foods Marketing Institute, Environmental Health Perspectives

In addition to cosmetic products, phthalates are added to plastic polymers and common household items such as toys, candles, vinyl flooring, garden hoses, air fresheners, paint, glue - even car dashes, and much more.

The *Department of Health and Human Services* and the *EPA* have classified phthalates as a probable human carcinogen and the *Centers for Disease Control* confirmed that humans can accumulate phthalates. When in our systems they can mimic estrogen, cause hormonal imbalances, as well as affect the thyroid, slow the metabolism, cause weight gain, loss of muscle mass in women, affect the size of the fetus and reduce the sperm count in men!!

Whether exposed via skin contact or inhaled, phthalates can cause allergies, asthma, sinus issues, headaches, rashes, and may even damage our kidneys, liver and lungs. Choose products that are noted as organic and unscented. If you like fragrance, safe scents are usually noted as essential oils, extracts and natural fragrance. Contact the manufacturer to be 100% sure the fragrance used is not a synthetic phthalate.

Your skin is like a sponge and absorbs just about anything you put on it.

How to Identify Phthalates

The word *phthalates* is often not placed on cosmetic and fragrance labels. I suggest contacting manufacturers to request the ingredients in your favorite perfumes, colognes, makeup and skin care products. The following list reveals a number of chemical names for phthalates: DEHP, butyl benzyl phthalate, di-n-butyl phthalate, mono-butyl phthalate, di-n-octyl phthalate, diethyl phthalate, dimethyl phthalate, mono-2-ethyl-5-hydroxyhexyl, mono-2-ethyl-5-oxohexyl, mono-2-ethylhexyl phthalate, mono-benzyl phthalate, mono-isobutyl phthalate, mono-ethyl phthalate, and mono-methyl phthalate.

Make a habit of avoiding products made with phthalates; especially those who are planning to become or are pregnant, or if going through hormonal changes such as menopause. Avoid all hair, body care, and household products that contain synthetic fragrances. Toss fragranced candles, room deodorizers, laundry and household cleansers that are made with synthetic fragrances. Choose fragrance-free products to be on the safe side or purchase products scented with *essential oils* and *extracts*. Make your own scented body products with safe, natural essential oils. See some of my favorite free beauty recipes at www.Youtube.com/user/BeautyGuru/videos. I've also noted some safe household cleaning recipes in the upcoming section.

Other Ingredients to Avoid

Below is a list of other questionable ingredients to look for on labels. Become a "label sleuth" to ensure that you and your family are using the safest products.

Petroleum found in cosmetics may cause dermatitis and are often contaminated with cancer-causing impurities. Petroleum can clog the pores, and may cause blackheads and dry skin with continued use.

Sodium lauryl sulfates (SLS), a foaming agent found in some shampoos, toothpastes and body washes dry out and strip the skin and hair of natural oils, allowing other chemicals to penetrate into the skin and muscles. A famous Hollywood hairdresser revealed to me that sodium lauryl sulfates are so strong they can remove rust from metal. SLS can dry the scalp is known to be one of the causes of falling hair.

Though not additives, **mercury, lead** and **cadmium** are the common elements found in household batteries. Be sure to wash your hands after handling them.

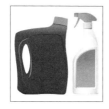

Age-Proofing Tip #13
Switch to Healthy Household Cleaners

Many household cleaning products including laundry detergent, bleach, fabric softener, dish soap, bathroom cleansers, floor products, and soap contain contaminants that are linked to cancer and lung issues. Inhaling these toxic agents affect our health and how we feel.

What's even more alarming is that federal laws don't require manufacturers of household cleaning products to disclose ingredients on their labels!

However, you can reduce exposure to harmful additives and other carcinogenic ingredients by choosing 'green' household cleaning products. They are readily available at health food and select grocery stores. Healthy cleaning products are noted as unscented, scented with essential oils, or listed as free of phosphates, dyes, phthalates (synthetic fragrances) and petroleum.

Safe Household Cleaning Brands

Some excellent and healthy brands of laundry detergent are **Seventh Generation® Natural Power Laundry Detergent and Chlorine-Free Bleach *Green Shield® Organic Laundry and Organic Fabric Softener *Trader Joe's® Liquid Laundry Detergent with Lavender Essential Oil *Bright Green® Laundry Detergent, Fabric Softener and Dish Washing Liquid *Eco® *Martha Stewart® *Bon Ami® *The Honest Company® *Whole Foods 365® Everyday Value® Laundry Detergent and 365® Stain Remover & Pre-wash.**

Visit EWG.org for more safe household products. The researchers painstakingly researched and tested over 2,000 household products and rated them for safety.

Environmental Working group (EWG.org) recently noted that *"Johnson & Johnson®, one of the world's largest personal care product companies announced a groundbreaking new initiative to reformulate many of its personal care products."* It's nice to know that many of the industry leaders in body care are now focusing on making healthier products. If we voice our opinions, hopefully Congress will pressure all manufacturers to make products that are free of harmful chemicals.

Make Your Own Household Cleaners

White distilled vinegar and baking soda are two of the most versatile, safe and cost effective household cleaners that do not harm our health. Use white vinegar as a fabric softener, bleach alternative and germ killer. Both vinegar and baking soda can be added to whites or colors to help brighten and prevent colors from running. This dynamic duo also deodorizes laundry. For those who are allergic to bleach **here's what you do:**

Pour 1 cup Heinz® white vinegar, 1 cup Arm & Hammer® baking soda and ½ cup 20 Mule Team® Borax in with the wash cycle.

I highly recommend spraying distilled white vinegar on counter tops, cutting boards and floor areas where animals eat, as a safe disinfectant. We have a Shark® floor steamer. Though it requires no soap we add ¼ cup vinegar to the water for additional disinfecting. See more laundry and cleaning tips below.

More cleaning uses for distilled white vinegar:
-clean off kitchen counter tops and cutting boards;
-wash fruits and vegetables;
-remove scents from used BPA-free plastic food storage containers;
-clean windows and mirrors;
-add to a floor steamer or into a mop bucket; and
-disinfect laundry.

More cleaning uses for baking soda:
-scrub sinks, toilets and bathroom tile;
-clean pots and pans;
-use as a drain cleaner; and
-laundry brightener and deodorizer.

TIP: Be sure to wear rubber gloves when doing housework. Keeping hands out of water can help prevent arthritis in hands and protect nails.

*To scrub sinks and remove soapy mildew in bathrooms **here's what you do:**

Spray vinegar on the surface, then sprinkle with a little baking soda, a squirt of natural phosphate-free dish soap and scrub with a Scotch Guard® non-scratch scrub sponge. Rinse afterwards.

*To scrub toilets, **here's what you do:**

Pour ½ cup baking soda, ½ cup white vinegar and a drop or two of natural phosphate-free dish soap into the toilet and scrub away. Allow the mixture to stay in the toilet until your next flush.

*To make a natural drain cleaner **here's what you do:**

Pour ½ cup Arm & Hammer® baking soda down the drain and top with 1 cup white vinegar. Let sit for an hour and then run HOT water down the drain.

*To make a window and mirror cleaner **here's what you do:**

Pour equal parts ½ vinegar and ½ water into a spray bottle.

*To clean pots and pans **here's what you do:**

Sprinkle with baking soda and a drop of phosphate-free, natural dish soap and scrub with a Scotch Guard® non-scratch scrub sponge.

*You'll love my healthy hand soap dispenser alternative. **Here's what you do:**

Instead of filling hand soap dispensers with commercial hand sanitizers, I use natural phosphate-free liquid dish soap fragranced with natural essential oils instead. Dish soap is economical too.

*To make a healthy air freshener **here's what you do:**

Pour 1 cup water into a spray bottle and add 10 drops rosemary or eucalyptus oil. Spray this healthy disinfectant around your home during cold or flu season or as a bathroom air deodorizer.

Alternative Laundry Tips:

*For whites **here's what you do:**

For a *full load* of whites, pour ½ cup 20 Mule Team® Borax or Arm & Hammer® baking soda, 1 cup chlorine-free bleach such as Bright White®, and your choice of laundry detergent for sensitive skin (free of perfume and dyes). I also recommend pouring your fabric softener in with the wash cycle. I like Bright White® perfume and dye-free fabric softener. It's scented with natural lavender extract. The little hint of lavender makes clothes smell fresh. White vinegar can also be used as a fabric softener.

*For colors **here's what you do:**

For a *full load* of colors, combine ½ cup 20 Mule Team® Borax or Arm & Hammer® baking soda, 1 cup Heinz® white distilled vinegar (prevents colors from fading), and your choice of laundry detergent for sensitive skin (free of perfume and dyes). I also recommend pouring your fabric softener in with the wash cycle. I like Bright White® perfume and dye-free fabric softener. It's scented with natural lavender extract. White vinegar can also be used as a fabric softener.

Hand Sanitizer Tip:

While on the go, instead of using commercial hand sanitizers that may contain parabens and phthalates, make your own. See my hand sanitizer recipe below. Use the wipes after handling money, restaurant menus, opening doors or any time on the go. The vinegar in this recipe kills many types of bacteria including e-coli. The wipes can be used to naturally disinfect hands and other surfaces. I even use them to wipe off the airport bins used to place shoes and personal items. Just think about it - dirty shoes are being placed in the *same* bins where we place our clothes, purses, belts, keys and laptops and become contaminated with millions of nasty germs. Yikes! Use the wipes to safely disinfect feet after walking barefoot through airport metal detectors and on airplane table trays and arm rests too. Enjoy my hand safe hand sanitizer recipe. **Here's what you do:**

Place 8-10 paraben and phthalate-free baby wipes such as Seventh Generation® or plain paper towels/napkins into a zipper lock sandwich bag. Add 2 tsp. Heinz® white distilled vinegar and keep the sealed bag in your purse.

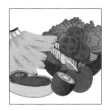

Age-Proofing Tip #14
Avoid Pesticides & Antibiotics in Food

The key to achieving good health is consuming fresh, pesticide-free foods. Thousands of scientific studies have proven that proper nutrition can provide longevity, long-term quality health and an uplifted mood. For wellbeing and balanced hormones, incorporate 'clean' foods such as antibiotic and hormone-free poultry, lean red meats, eggs, dairy and pesticide-free organic fruits and vegetables. Grass fed beef is known to be lower in fat. Choose high protein grains, nuts, unsaturated oils, and low glycemic fruits to decrease the risk of hormonal imbalances, prevent insulin resistance, moodiness, blood sugar spikes, weight gain, and disease. There's nothing like the experience of eating delicious, healthy foods. When we eat healthy, we become energized.

For hormonal stability during and after pregnancy, monthly menstruation, and all stages of menopause, consuming healthy 'clean' foods can help improve our mood and reduce irritability, hot flashes or night sweats. Menopause is a natural passage of life. You'll have a much easier time of it by choosing foods marked organic, or free of hormones and antibiotics. In addition, minimize or avoid eating processed, cured and smoked meats, trans-fats such as margarine or lard, deep fried foods, and those that list artificial ingredients on their labels. Artificial ingredients are difficult for the body to digest. They hinder our weight loss goals and cause myriad health concerns.

Organic, pesticide-free produce and antibiotic and hormone-free meats, eggs, and dairy are readily available in regular supermarket chains and are now more reasonably priced. Read about super foods in **Age-Proofing Tip #53** and when you have time, check out Worldshealthiestfoods.com for information on organic foods, nutritional values and healthy recipes.

Cleaning Fruits and Veggies

*If you do not have access to pesticide-free produce, purchase a veggie wash such as **Natural Environne® Fruit and Vegetable Wash**. It is a safe, yet powerful cleanser that removes pesticides, waxes and chemicals. Many reports suggest avoiding *porous* fruits such as strawberries and raspberries as pesticides are extremely difficult to wash off their surfaces. Many *non-organic* apples are known to be heavily laden with pesticides, so it is best to peel them.

*To clean fruits and vegetables, whether organic or not, an economical cleaner is white vinegar. It even kills ecoli that is often found in fruit rinds such as cantaloupes, lemons and oranges.

*Grapefruit seed extract can be diluted with water and used to wash fruits, vegetables, clean kitchen counters, cutting boards, toothbrushes, and more. It's even used as a natural preservative in many natural skin care products. It prevents bacterial growth. In fact, I use grapefruit seed extract in some of my beauty recipes. I'm a fan of **NutriBiotic® *Original Grapefruit Seed Extract***. Follow the directions on the bottle for many health-safe disinfecting and anti-bacterial purposes.

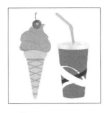

Age-Proofing Tip #15
Avoid Artificial Sweeteners

Avoid artificial sweeteners especially if you've been having difficulty losing weight. If you think that drinking diet sodas and foods laden with artificial sweeteners can help with weight loss, the following facts reveal otherwise.

-*The Journal of the American Medical Association* reported, "Although low-calorie sweeteners are a dietary staple for many individuals trying to maintain or lose weight, an emerging body of evidence suggests these substances offer little help to dieters and may even help promote weight gain."

-The *National Institute of Health* and *University of Miami* researchers report that drinking more than two diet sodas a day is associated with heart disease, stroke, and may increase the risk of developing type 2 diabetes.

-Doctor Alicia Stanton, international speaker and author of 'The *Complete Idiot's Guide to Hormone Weight Loss'* notes, "The way these zero-calorie artificial sweeteners lead to weight gain is by tricking the brain into expecting more calories, thereby promoting desire for sweet foods. Aspartame breaks down into methyl alcohol, a chemical that is associated with a number of side effects, including decreased vision, seizures, migraines, memory loss, irritability and hyperactivity. Sucralose has been linked to migraines and low thyroid." Find out more about artificial sweeteners in Dr. Stanton's popular book, available at Amazon.com and select bookstores.

Healthy, Tasty Sweeteners

Diet foods and drinks that contain artificial sweeteners make us crave the foods we want to avoid! Better health-wise, natural choices are xylitol, stevia, organic raw agave, or honey. See a brief description of each natural sweetener below:

Stevia is a natural zero calorie herb grown in South America. It's a healthy sugar substitute that tastes very sweet, though it doesn't cause dental cavities. Stevia is known to regulate blood sugar, lower triglycerides and blood pressure and is a digestive aid too. Stevia is about four times sweeter than sugar so do not measure it out like sugar. You need very little. I sprinkle it into hot or cold beverages. It's recommended for those with weight loss needs and those challenged with diabetes or hypoglycemia. One tsp. = 0 calories

Xylitol is a healthy natural sweetener that tastes and looks like real sugar, but does not raise blood sugar. It is a low glycemic, gluten-free, non-GMO, 100% natural sugar alternative that measures, looks and tastes like real sugar but is lower in calories. Those prone to dental cavities, yeast infections, and diabetes can safely use xylitol. It prevents tooth decay, bad breath, and yeast buildup. I use xylitol for making guilt-free desserts and in hot green tea. It's heat-stable for baking and cooking too. I like the brand XyloSweet®, available at health food stores.
One tsp. = 9.5 calories

Organic raw agave is a natural sugar substitute that tastes sweeter than honey, so you require less of it. Agave is gluten-free and low-glycemic so it digests more slowly than sugar, preventing spikes in insulin. The anti-inflammatory properties of agave may be a better choice for those with inflammatory challenges such as lupus, arthritis, fibromyalgia or MS. Many anti-aging experts claim that sugar causes inflammation which contributes to pain and aged looking skin. **TIP:** Make my wheat-free, high protein pancakes and top them with agave instead of maple syrup. **WARNING:** If pregnant, do not use agave. It may cause miscarriage.
One tsp. = 20 calories

Raw honey contains many healthy properties such as vitamin A, B, beta carotene, minerals and natural antibiotic properties. It's not quite as sweet as raw agave yet sweeter than sugar. Honey may be linked to better memory and longer lifespan. Read more about honey in **Age-Proofing Tip #53 - Super Foods.** I like to add a little raw honey to lemon tea during cold winter months as a cold or flu preventative. **WARNING:** Honey should not be given to babies under the age of three. It contains spores that are not safe for infants.
One tsp. = 20 calories

According to a *Nutrition Action Health Letter*, Splenda® and Truvia® appear to be safe. See sources for products listed in **Safe, Effective Face & Body Product Suggestions.**

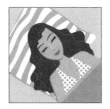

Age-Proofing Tip #16
Importance of Rejuvenating Sleep

Sleep is rejuvenating. Did you know that without sufficient sleep the body ages even faster? Getting eight hours of uninterrupted nightly sleep helps the body to renew and heal itself. Many sleep studies have proven that restful sleep can improve our health, both physically and emotionally, and naturally increases our production of human growth hormone (HGH). HGH is produced by the pituitary gland. It helps reduce fat stored in our cells and combats many signs of aging. The good news is, HGH can be increased naturally and without the need of dangerous, costly HGH injections as you will read below.

Other Reasons to Get More Sleep

Hormone health specialist, Dr. Alicia Stanton, notes that lack of sleep interferes with fat burning too. Sleeplessness stimulates hunger and triggers insulin resistance which interferes with how the body metabolizes fat, resulting in weight gain. Further studies conclude that getting less than seven to eight hours of uninterrupted sleep can double your risk of catching a cold or flu. According to a *University of Berkeley* study, disrupted sleep reduces our energy during the day and can cause a 60% increase in anxiety and stress. Sleep deprivation causes loss of concentration, affects the immune system, impairs motor skills and causes mood swings. Another recent study revealed that overweight post-menopausal women with breast cancer, experience higher hormone levels that trigger more aggressive breast cancer tumor growth if they sleep <u>less than seven hours nightly</u>.

Signs of Low HGH

By age 30, our natural production of HGH dramatically declines which can cause many individuals to look and feel older than their actual age. Signs of low HGH are increased abdominal fat on the stomach, muffin tops/love handles, loss of elasticity and sagging skin, wrinkles, loss of muscle tone, grey hair, cellulite, low energy and libido, mood swings, depression, impaired vision, high cholesterol, thickening and hardening of the arteries and plaque formation.

Sufficient sleep and weight resistance exercise stimulates HGH production. Read more about weight resistance in **Age-Proofing Tip #57.** Below are several tips that can help induce restful sleep and naturally increase HGH production.

How to Catch More Zees

*Our bodies release HGH several times a day. However, its highest spike occurs at the *beginning* of our sleep cycle. For this reason, **calming ourselves prior to bedtime** is paramount. This ensures falling asleep faster. Read a book, pray or meditate.

***Do not watch violent or disturbing TV shows**, movies or the evening news prior to sleep. They cause anxiety which prevents falling asleep faster. Watch a comedy instead.

***Avoid caffeine after 3:00 p.m.** and take vitamins with breakfast and lunch to ensure better sleep. Supplements such as resveratrol and omega 3s can be taken at dinner without disturbing rest. Read more about the age-defying and weight loss benefits of resveratrol and omega 3 in **Age-Proofing Tip #51 - My Favorite Supplements for Women**.

*Studies have proven that the phytochemicals in **hot black tea** encourage restful sleep. I like to drink Lipton® and earl grey tea approximately two hours before bedtime. I also recommend drinking hot or iced herbal teas such as hibiscus, chamomile or valerian root. They are all calming, zero-calorie beverages.

***Tryptophan** is an essential amino acid found in many foods. It triggers the nervous system to raise serotonin levels which regulates anxiety, insomnia, moodiness and even depression. Include tryptophan-rich foods at dinner time to help induce a more relaxing sleep. They include turkey, tofu, shrimp, chicken, tuna, cod, salmon, soybeans, pumpkin seeds, spinach, asparagus, green beans, lentils, or quinoa. See more calming foods in **Age-Proofing Tip #9.**

*Unlike prescription drugs, **5-HTP** is a non-addictive, drug-free amino acid derived from plants. 5-HTP signals messages through the nervous system promoting a positive, uplifted mood throughout the day and a calmer, rested feeling at night. It's a natural feel-good neurotransmitter! Another bonus of 5-HTP is it helps curb appetite. I like Natrol® brand because it's time released. I take 100 mg of 5-HTP nightly to ensure a restful sleep. For those with a busy daily schedule, 5-HTP can be a very beneficial daily supplement because it can help maintain calmness. Other brands of 5-HTP are combined with stress-busting B-vitamins.

***Magnesium** is an excellent night time supplement that can address anxiety, fear, moodiness, insomnia, depression, and brain fog. Magnesium citrate (300 mg) is recommended because it is readily absorbed. The other benefits of taking this supplement nightly is that it calms muscles, reduces restless or twitching legs, induces deep relaxation and can even halt teeth grinding. Grinding teeth while asleep is a sign of stress. In addition, if you're challenged with constipation, magnesium helps loosen bowels by morning. Magnesium is found in dairy products and in foods such as pumpkin seeds, spinach, swiss chard, sunflower seeds, figs and sesame seeds. **NOTE:** Magnesium can interfere with some medications so check with your doctor on the best time to take it.

*Stress causes an increase in the production of cortisol and insulin which can result in weight gain and extra inches around the midriff and hips. What many women don't know is that excessive cortisol production keeps us awake at night too! Not to worry! **Melatonin** can help. We all naturally produce the hormone melatonin which induces sleep and improves memory. As we age, melatonin production slows down. However, the good news is, when taken as a supplement *20 minutes before bed*, melatonin *shuts off* cortisol production, allowing a good night's sleep, better memory and more success with weight loss goals. Taking a melatonin supplement will not disrupt the body's natural production of it. In additional, melatonin is a powerful antioxidant and anti-depressant that regulates the immune system. So it's HIGHLY recommended for those who feel or look older, are stressed, challenged with insomnia, weight gain, moodiness, or brain fog. Those with a history of Alzheimer's disease take melatonin because it increases their learning ability. Instead of taking sleeping pills, natural melatonin is an excellent alternative sleep enhancer. **NOTE:** Melatonin can react with some medications, such as monoamine oxidize inhibitors (MOI's). Also do not take this supplement during the day as it causes drowsiness.

*Bright lights block melatonin production. With this in mind, do not watch TV in bed and turn all lights off in your bedroom.

***Gaba** contains natural, safe rejuvenating properties, increases concentration and can reduce stress. It helps naturally increase HGH (human growth hormone) production which substantially decreases once we hit age 40.

***Dream Water**® is a drug-free, all-natural sleep and relaxation beverage that is packaged much like those energy shot bottles. However, it does the opposite. Dream Water® combines 5-HTP, melatonin and gaba to help reduce stress, induce relaxation and sleep. It's zero calories, all natural and sweetened with natural stevia.

*By the time we reach our mid-30's our bodies produce less natural HGH. Amino acids play an essential role in building protein and maintaining hormone health especially for those who are feeling or looking older than their years. ***Meditropin**® is an effervescent drink mix that can energize, nourish, repair and rejuvenate the body. It is rich in amino acids that help naturally stimulate HGH production but is *not a steroid or HGH.* Meditropin® can help nourish the adrenals and pituitary glands for hormonal support. When combined with a low carbohydrate diet, it can help increase energy, provide a more restful sleep, and improve muscle tone, increase libido and much more. It is used worldwide. Find out more information and read the health constraints and ingredients at www.nutraceutics.com. They recommend taking the product for three consecutive months five nights a week. Check with your health care professional before ordering this product. This product is not recommended for vegetarians or vegans as it contains porcine and fish.

*The challenge of **nighttime acid reflux** can cause sleepless-ness. Reclining after eating dinner is one reason. However, tak-ing 1 tbsp. of **apple cider vinegar** mixed with a glass of water approximately one hour after your last meal of the day can help speed digestion and prevent acid reflux for a better night's sleep.

In addition to sleep, weight resistance exercise and eating low-carbohydrate foods can help our bodies produce more HGH. Bottom line is that increased HGH production rejuvenates us. I will outline more about how food and exercise can affect HGH production on upcoming pages.

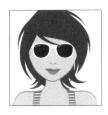

Age-Proofing Tip #17
Safe Sun Exposure

As we age, wrinkles appear on our faces due to free radical exposure and habitual facial expressions. Over time, the skin's ability to heal itself slows as does cell regeneration and the production of collagen, elastin and hyaluronic acid, resulting in aged-looking skin. Smoking, stress and gravity add to the lines, wrinkles, dark spots, and sagging skin that many women experience by age 40. But THE worst culprit of all is exposure to the sun! The sun's damaging UV rays cause oxidation resulting in wrinkles, age-spots, uneven skin tone and several forms of skin cancer. Did you know that skin damage can start after just ONE minute of sun exposure? Below are some important new sun facts and skin saver tips that you need to know.

*The sun is responsible for 75% of wrinkles on our faces, as well as age spots on the hands and chest area.

*Tanning beds are NOT a safer way to tan and should be avoided. UCLA Dermatology research reveals that those who use tanning beds are at higher risk for developing skin cancers such as basal cell carcinoma, malignant melanoma and squamous cell carcinoma (the most common type of skin cancer). In addition, tanning beds may be linked to macular degeneration.

*The sun's UVB rays penetrate the epidermis (outer layer of skin) causing sunburns and tans. They speed skin aging and cause squamous cell carcinoma. When caught early, this type of skin cancer is treatable.

*The sun's UVA rays penetrate deep down into the dermis (the second layer of skin), where collagen is formed or breaks down. UVA rays cause skin aging, wrinkles, loss of elasticity, dark spots and more serious cellular damage that can result in both basal cell carcinoma and melanoma cancers. Melanoma, the more serious of the two, can rapidly spread throughout skin tissue and can be deadly if not treated early.

*UV damage is known to cause eye issues such as cataracts, macular degeneration and deeper wrinkle formation around the eyes.

*Ears and toes are two of the most common areas for skin cancer to appear.

*Adults in their 30s are now the highest demographic with more cases of skin cancer being reported. Their rates are far higher than individuals in their 50s - as was once the case.

*Even on cloudy days, the majority of ultraviolet rays are reflected by cement (walking on sidewalks), sand (beach), snow (skiing or snowboarding), and water (swimming in pools, lakes and oceans). When I was a guest beauty expert on Sirius XM's The Dermatology Show with Dr. Day, she mentioned that some of the worst sunburns she treated were had by those who spent hours out on a cloudy day, without sunscreen.

Skin Saver Tips

The types of foods we eat and the products we apply onto our skin can be age-proofing and lower our risk of skin cancer. Free radicals such as sun and pollution cause oxidation - attacking our cells. We can neutralize oxidation and help protect our skin from harmful UV rays by incorporating the following age-defying skin saver tips.

*Consume colorful antioxidant rich fruits and veggies. They are rich in caratenoids and flavonoids which provide the skin with natural sun protection from the inside out. In addition, flavonoids prevent the destruction of collagen. These powerful antioxidants accumulate in our skin, attack harmful free radicals, lower the risk of sun damage, prevent inflammation and oxidation, and can even lower the risk of cataracts. Your skin will look younger and you'll feel healthier by eating nourishing, colorful, fresh organic produce.

*Green tea offers myriad age-proofing and health support. It contains anti-inflammatory agents that fight free radicals and prevent loss of glutathione (a natural detoxifier found in every cell of the body) which protects our health. Both drinking green tea and applying topical green tea products can improve collagen production for firm, more youthful-looking, hydrated skin. Green tea provides additional UV protection from the sun as well as anti-microbial properties that help keep blemishes in check. Read more benefits of green tea in **Age-Proofing Tip #51 - My Favorite Supplements for Women.**

*In my previous books I've recommended applying a 30 SPF facial sunscreen each morning. However, when discussing new SPF regulations with Dr. Linda Miles, a highly respected leader in holistic medicine and natural skin care formulations, she revealed that applying an SPF 15 sunscreen is plenty of protection for normal, everyday wear. SPF is the abbreviation for sun protection factor. It is the international standard for measuring the effectiveness of sunscreen. For example, by applying an SPF 15 sunscreen, you can safely be exposed to the sun's UV rays 15 times longer than if wearing no sunscreen. Dr. Miles suggested that the only time we need to apply a higher SPF sunscreen (30) is when we plan to spend several hours out in the sun. As far as everyday shopping, working and walking, SPF 15 is sufficient.

*Since the new sunscreen FDA regulations came into play in 2012, I began my mission to uncover a paraben and phthalate-free broad spectrum UVA/UVB SPF 15 facial sunscreen. I tested over a dozen healthy sunscreens, but with little satisfaction. Most were too thick, too greasy or dry-looking on the skin. They looked too white and were impossible to cover with makeup. In addition, they were overpriced at $35 and over. I almost gave up hope but I stayed on focused on my mission and I am happy to report, that after months of testing various brands, I finally found a terrific, cost-effective facial sunscreen! It's called **Evenly Radiant Day Crème** with SPF 15. It offers plenty of UVA/UVB protection for everyday wear, it doesn't leave a thick or white film, and contains nourishing antioxidants and natural skin bleaching agents. It's hydrating but doesn't feel greasy. Every person I've recommended it to - loves it. Men and teens included. Plus, it's suitable for all skin types and ideal under all types of makeup - including powder mineral makeup! I love it too. ☺ My skin looks dewy, fresh and youthful. When I'm out in public, many women ask me what I use on my skin. **Here's what I do:**

In the morning, after cleansing and toning, I apply De-Aging Solution or Ultimate Age-Proofing Complex. Then, I apply Evenly Radiant Day Crème (SPF 15) on top. I wait two minutes for the sunscreen to settle and apply my powder mineral makeup.

*New sun protection guidelines require that all sunscreens, even those labeled as high as SPF 50, require re-application every two hours when outdoors. For body application, I recommend **Natural Sun® Green Tea Sunscreen SPF 30+** by Aubrey Organics with 12% zinc oxide, 5.6% titanium dioxide green tea and plant-based emollients. It provides excellent coverage that's not as white as other broad spectrum sunscreens. Because it's micronized, it doesn't penetrate into the skin and muscles, thus considered safer than sunscreens made with nano-particles. Another brand that I recommend for body wear and longer spells outdoors is **Neutrogena® Pure & Free Liq-**

uid Daily Sun Block™. It contains 100% naturally sourced minerals, free of fragrance, dyes, and irritating chemical ingredients. See where to purchase these and other healthy sunscreen choices in **Safe, Effective Face & Body Product Suggestions.**

*Broad spectrum UVB + UVA ingredients include zinc oxide and titanium dioxide. They create a physical barrier, filtering both types of rays when applied on the skin. They are made of up natural minerals that refract the harmful rays away from skin and do not absorb. This prevents allergic reactions, break outs and disruption of hormones.

*Wear sunscreen on cloudy days too.

*In addition to face and body, be sure to apply sunscreen on ears and toes. If wearing open-toed shoes or sitting on a boat for hours at a time, re-apply sunscreen on top of feet every two hours or switch to running shoes for full foot protection. Also wear a wide brimmed hat to protect ears.

*When outdoors wear long sleeves, gloves, and a wide-brimmed visor or hat to provide a physical block from the sun.

*Mineral powder makeup provides some additional healthy sun protection though it is recommended to always apply sunscreen first. Mineral makeup is anti-microbial so it can help prevent breakouts. It's great for all skin types especially those with acne or blemish-prone skin. See more helpful tips about acne in **Age-Proofing Tip #22 - Universal Skin Care Regimens** (Acne or Blemish-Prone Skin) and **Age-Proofing Tip #24 - Blemish & Acne Prevention.**

*Damaging UV rays can penetrate through windshield glass. To protect hands from sun's UV rays wear cotton gloves when driving. My hands still look young and free of sun spots because I wear gloves whenever outdoors or driving. And I wear a long sleeved cotton shirt whenever in my car. This protects my arms, décolletage, and neck from UV rays coming through the windshield. **TIP:** Keep a shirt in your car at all times. When driving toward the sun, place a shirt on backwards so the collar covers the neck and chest as well as your arms.

*Protect eyes by wearing polarized sunglasses when outdoors or driving. They help block the eyes from harmful UV rays, which can prevent cataracts later in life.

*Avoid UV rays when they are most intense - between the hours of 10 a.m. and 3 p.m. If you jog, walk a dog, or play outdoor sports, do so either early in the morning or later in the evening to avoid the sun's strongest rays.

*After a day out in the sun, apply a hydrating body lotion that contains antioxidants, vitamin C, and green tea as they provide additional skin soothing and anti-inflammatory properties. **Skinlasting Super Hydrator** is an all-natural spray that is free of petroleum, paraben and fragrance. It contains green tea, vitamin C, and hydrating hyaluronic acid so it's a wonderful post-sun and post-shower body hydrator and gentle exfoliant. **Hydrating Hyaluronic Mist** is another good choice. Find both products listed under Hyaluronic Acid Products in **Safe, Effective Face & Body Product Suggestions.**

*Another post-sun choice that costs just pennies is organic food grade coconut oil. When applied sparingly and massaged into skin, coconut oil's lauric acid offers skin healing, and antibacterial properties. Coconut oil protects the skin from UV rays while it provides a nice moisturizing base under the thicker zinc/titanium oxide body sunscreens which makes for easier removal of the sunscreen when showering. Coconut oil can be applied on the body or face and does not clog pores. Read more about coconut oil in **Age-Proofing Tip #26 - Beauty Oils.**

*Once a year, see your dermatologist for a complete skin check, and each month examine your skin for changes in moles or new ones that pop up.

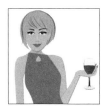

Age-Proofing Tip #18
Limit Alcohol & Do Not Smoke

Consuming excessive amounts of alcohol dehydrates the skin and affects the skin's elasticity especially when asleep. Alcohol slows the blood flow that repairs skin while asleep. It also affects the production of the sleep hormone melatonin. With this in mind it is best to limit use of alcohol to three glasses a week. Red wine in moderation is okay. Drinking hard liquor is known to increase the risk of breast cancer.

For great health and younger-looking skin - do not smoke. Besides being a huge health hazard, smoking ages the face, body and hands, causes broken blood vessels, enlarged pores, pigmentation spots, lines around the mouth, crow's feet, a dull complexion, loss of elasticity in skin and wrinkles! Do your best to stop smoking. Try chewing gum or wear smokers' patches, which are formulated to help eliminate dependence on cigarettes. Hypnosis is another alternative that has helped many individuals.

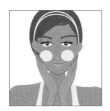

Age-Proofing Tip #19
Exfoliate Skin

As we age, skin cell regeneration slows down to about every 48 days resulting in dull, dry and mature-looking skin. To speed cell regeneration, exfoliating the skin provides transforming, age-defying results. Exfoliation brightens and evens the complexion by loosening dull, dry skin cells and allows fresh new cells to surface. Collagen and elastin production increases resulting in thicker, younger-looking skin. In addition, exfoliation reduces age spots, fine lines, acne and blemishes scars, and unclogs pores.

How and When to Exfoliate Skin

Exfoliate skin two to three times per week <u>only</u>. Doing so more often can cause excessively thin, fragile skin. When exfoliating be sure to include temples and jowls, jaw line, neck, chest, hands, arms, elbows, knees, and thighs to keep skin looking more firm and youthful. After just a few weeks of regular exfoliation, you'll begin to notice thicker skin, less protruding veins on the temples, a tighter jaw line and jowls, firmer skin on the neck, and reduced age spots on hands, chest and face.

Below I've outlined a variety of exfoliants. They include creams, cleansers, liquids, masks, enzymes, scrubs and special tools. Find the products noted in **Safe, Effective Face & Body Product Suggests.**

Types of Exfoliants - Acids

Exfoliating acids naturally occur in fruit, milk, plants and sugar, and are added to creams, masks, peels, cleansers, lotions and sprays.

Lactic, glycolic and **alpha hydroxy acids (AHA)** exfoliate and hydrate the skin therefore are more suitable for those who require more moisture (ages 35 and up). AHA's reduce milia, clogged pores, dry or dull-looking skin and can help fade superficial scars. Find lactic, glycolic and alpha hydroxy acids in a variety of creams, peels and cleansers. Choose an AHA cream that is pH balanced such as ***Evenly Radiant Overnight Peel.*** It's inexpensive too. Read more about exfoliating cleansers below.

Citric acid is fruit based and can help 'bleach' the skin, fade age spots and superficial acne scars. It can be used by those

55

with normal, dry, mature, dull or uneven skin. My yogurt & lemon mask recipe below, combines lactic and citric acid. It even provides a skin-tightening, yet hydrating, face-lifting effect. **Here's what you do:**

Combine 2 tbsp. plain yogurt, 1 tsp. fresh lemon juice and 1 capsule hyaluronic acid (80 mg) and mix well. Apply mixture on clean face. Leave on for 20 minutes until the mask dries. Wash of with tepid water.

Beta hydroxy acid (BHA) includes salicylic acid or **benzoyl peroxide.** These exfoliants help reduce clogged pores such as whiteheads and blackheads. In addition, they can help reduce milia and prevent inflammation and bacteria associated with acne and blemish breakouts. Salicylic acid is found in peels, topical 'spot' treatments and facial cleansers. A paraben and phthalate-free salicylic acid cleanser I recommend is *Beyond Clean*. Benzoyl peroxide cleansers and topical spot treatments are available at all drug stores.

Retinol (AKA retinoids) is a powerful and more costly exfoliating option. It is usually prescribed by a dermatologist or skin care specialist and recommended to those with severe sun damage, uneven pigmentation, deep wrinkles, acne or blemish-breakouts, milia or facial scars. Use retinol in moderation as it can cause redness and dry, flaky skin. If you are experiencing thinning, fragile, dry or peeling skin, cut back the application to one or two times a week. This allows time for fresh cells to re-build and thicken the skin. *O24U Hyperoxygenated Gel* contains retinol (vitamin A). Apply it nightly on acne or blemish spots using a cotton swab, or on the entire face once weekly as a gentle, peeling mask. **NOTE**: Do not use retinol if planning to become, or are pregnant as vitamin A may cause birth defects.

Enzyme Peels are derived from fruits. They offer a gentle, yet effective skin exfoliating mask alternative for all skin types, including those with inflammation, rosacea or sensitive skin. Fruit enzymes gently dissolve dead surface layers, improve skin texture, firm the skin, remove impurities, help heal blemishes, brighten and even skin tone, and are rich in vitamins and minerals. My pumpkin mask enzyme peel is suitable for all skin types. Spas charge about $65 to $85 for an enzyme peel. Make your own pumpkin enzyme peel for $3. **Here's what you do:**

Combine 2 tbsp. plain pumpkin and 1 tbsp. honey or plain yogurt. Apply on clean skin for 20 minutes. Then rinse mask off with tepid water.

See a variety of facial masks in **More Beauty Recipes**.

NOTE: FDA studies have revealed that those who use hydroxy and glycolic acid products are more prone to sun sensitivity and UV damage. The same goes for retinoids. Be sure to apply daily SPF 15 broad spectrum sunscreen to protect against UV skin damage. While outdoors for long periods of time, re-apply sunscreen every two hours.

Exfoliating Cleansers

For those with sensitive, sun-damaged, mature/dry skin as well as those challenged with acne or rosacea, consider using a cream or liquid cleansing exfoliant, instead of a scrub. Choose cleansers that contain glycolic or salicylic acid such as *Glycolic Cleanser* **with marine plant extracts,** or *Beyond Clean* with salicylic acid and zinc to gently exfoliate without irritating the skin. Both are free of color, parabens, and synthetic phthalate/fragrance.

Exfoliating Liquids

Lactic acid in milk is a gentle, yet highly effective skin exfoliant. In addition, the fat in milk hydrates the skin. Take a milk bath once a week. It's suitable for all skin types. **Here's what you do:**

Pour a gallon of cold milk into a *hot* tub of water and soak for 20 minutes. Then rinse and pat skin dry.

I recommend applying a natural lactic acid-based body spray/mist after bathing. One that I personally use and have shared with thousands of women is *Skinlasting Super Hydrator*. It's an all-natural, paraben, phthalate, petroleum, dye and fragrance-free hydrating spray that contains vitamin C and green tea for UV protection, hyaluronic acid for hydration, lactic acid for exfoliation, and non-pore clogging vegetable glycerin. It was developed by a dermatologist for all skin types including those with mature, extremely dry or chicken bump skin. It can also benefit those with eczema, psoriasis, diabetic skin or dry post-chemotherapy skin conditions. Some senior tennis players report that it keeps their legs and arms looking more firm and smooth. Women who live in sunny or dry climates can't say enough good things about this natural hydrating body spray. **TIP:** Spray Skinlasting in your hand and apply it on neck, chest, arms, legs, hands and feet after showering.

Exfoliating Scrubs

NOTE: Scrub exfoliants are NOT recommended for those with rosacea or sensitive skin. Scrubs are best suited for individuals with normal, dry, mature, clogged or oily skin.

My baking soda scrub costs just pennies and is a quick, effective way to exfoliate both face and body. **Here's what you do:**

For <u>facial</u> exfoliation, cleanse skin. While face is still wet, grab a handful of baking soda and gently scrub skin in a circular motion. Then rinse. Follow with an antioxidant or peptide-rich lotion or serum.

For <u>body</u> exfoliation, apply baking soda on a wet face cloth and gently scrub in a circular motion from neck down to feet while in the shower. Or combine a handful of baking soda with a few pumps of liquid body wash and scrub skin.

An alternative scrub product that I personally use and have recommended to many individuals over the years is cost-effective **Microdermabrasion Scrub**. It's a paraben and phthalate-free paste made with volcanic sand, dead sea salt and other natural ingredients. It's a very powerful, salon skin treatment alternative. I apply a small amount of scrub onto clean skin using a gentle circular motion. To prevent the scrub from getting into my eyes, I apply the scrub on *dry skin* - not wet. Several women have reported that after using this scrub they no longer pay for costly professional microdermabrasion treatments. After just three uses, they achieve satisfying results.

NOTE: See more face and body exfoliation recipes in **More Beauty Recipes.**

Exfoliating Tools - Dry Brushing

Japanese women swear by dry brushing as an effective skin exfoliation method. Dry brushes are made with natural bristles and cost under $10 at most beauty supply, health food and drug stores. **Here's what you do:**

Prior to showering, dry brush each area in upward semi-circles for two minutes or until the skin turns slightly pink. If you don't have time to dry brush prior to showering, exfoliate body in the shower with a loofa.

See where to find these tools and products noted in **Safe, Effective Face & Body Product Suggests.** .

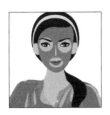

Age-Proofing Tip #20
Apply a Weekly Facial Mask

If you don't have the time or budget to indulge in a professional spa treatment, why not make your own mask using common foods and condiments found right in your home? Below are 10 effective facial masks for many skin types and challenges. Check with your physician before trying new ingredients or products. Use the recipes at your own risk.

RECIPE #1
Pumpkin Exfoliator (acne prone, rosacea, sensitive and all other skin types)

When making a pumpkin pie, save a little canned pumpkin to make this fast and effective recipe. The enzymes in pumpkin are beneficial to those who can't use scrubs. They gently exfoliate skin, unplug clogged pores, smooth fine lines, and brighten and calm tender or acne-prone skin. Pumpkin is a fruit, rich in carotene, pantothenic acid, potassium, magnesium, vitamin C and E and skin healing enzymes.

Ingredients:
3 tbsp. plain canned pumpkin
1 tsp. honey
1 tbsp. plain yogurt or cream

Combine ingredients in a glass bowl and stir to a paste. Apply on clean skin. Leave on for 20 minutes. Rinse off with tepid water.

RECIPE #2
Chlorophyll Firming Face Mask

Chlorophyll is rich in alguronic acid which is known to stimulate elastin production in the skin. According to a northern California biotechnology company, it may be more effective than retinol for exfoliating the skin. This facial mask helps firm and even skin tone.

Ingredients:
1 chlorophyll capsule (50 mg)
1 tsp. squalane or olive oil
1 tbsp. plain yogurt

Combine ingredients and apply mask on clean skin. Leave on for 30 minutes. Rinse off with tepid water.

RECIPE #3
Carrot Hydrator (dry skin)

Carrots nourish and hydrate dry skin. They are rich in carotene, copper and vitamin C & E to help moisturize dull, dehydrated skin.

Ingredients:
½ medium cooked, mashed carrot
1 tbsp. honey or plain yogurt
1 tbsp. oats

Combine ingredients in a bowl and apply mask onto clean skin.
Leave on for 30 minutes. Rinse off with tepid water.

RECIPE #4
Acorn Squash Rejuvenator (not for those with rosacea)

Acorn squash contains antioxidants, minerals and vitamins
that are essential for healthy, beautiful skin. Rich in omega
fats, carotene and vitamins A and C, this mask brightens and
firms aging skin.

Ingredients:
⅓ cup of mashed, cooked acorn squash
2 tbsp. olive oil
1 tbsp. ground almond meal

Apply on clean skin. Leave on for 20 minutes. Rinse off with
tepid water.

RECIPE #5
Apple Age-Spot Reducer (age spots, melasma and fine lines)

Malic acid in apples, lemon juice and turmeric are natural,
highly effective skin lighteners and brighteners. Apples are rich
in vitamin A, B, C, K, biotin and pantothenic acid.

Ingredients:
1 cored apple
2 tbsp. honey
1 tsp. fresh lemon juice
¼ tsp. spice turmeric

Place a raw apple in a blender or food processor until finely
chopped. Place blended apple in a bowl and add remaining ingredients. Apply on clean skin and leave on for 30 minutes.
Rinse off with tepid water.

RECIPE #6
Vitamin C Skin Brightening Mask (normal, dry or mature skin)

Ascorbic acid is a water soluble form of vitamin C (AKA L-ascorbic acid). When added to a facial cream or oil product, it can make a powerful skin brightening and pore refining mask. However, you must apply it immediately as this type of vitamin C loses its efficacy quickly. Every application must be made fresh. Ascorbic acid is not recommended for those with sensitive skin. See below for more information on how to make this recipe for sensitive skin.

If you have sensitive skin, you can make this recipe with ascorbyl palmitate, a fat soluble form of vitamin C (AKA vitamin C-ester). This form of vitamin C is gentler and more stable than ascorbic acid. Vitamin C-ester penetrates into cells and can help protect the skin from UV damage. See my favorite skin brightening vitamin C mask recipe below:

Ingredients:
¼ tsp. ascorbic acid powder or ascorbic palmitate powder
1 tsp. emu oil or squalane oil

Combine the ingredients and apply on clean skin. Leave on for 30 minutes. Rinse off with tepid water.

RECIPE #7
Acne Scar Eraser

This acne and scar reducing recipe is super effective. An added bonus of this mask is that it provides an instant skin-tightening and face-lifting effect that lasts for hours! The lactic acid in the yogurt exfoliates and the citric acid in the lemon juice gently bleaches the scars and brightens the skin tone.

Ingredients:
1 tbsp. fresh lemon juice
2 tbsp. plain yogurt

Combine the ingredients and apply the mixture on clean skin. Allow to dry for 20-30 minutes. Rinse off with tepid water.

RECIPE #8
Sunburned Skin Calmer

The vitamin A in pumpkin provides skin healing enzymes that reduce redness and gently calm skin. Honey is a natural humectant with skin soothing and antibacterial/antibiotic properties that speed heal tender, red, burned or irritated skin.

Ingredients:
1 50 mg capsule Pycnogenol® (antioxidant)
2 tbsp. plain canned pumpkin
1 tsp. honey

Break open the capsule, combine it with the remaining ingredients and apply on clean skin. Leave on for 30 minutes. Rinse off with tepid water.

RECIPE #9
Chocolate Antioxidant Mask

The beauty of chocolate is that it's high in antioxidants. Oats hydrate and calm skin, dairy gently exfoliates and brightens skin, and honey is a humectant that offers skin soothing and healing antibiotic properties.

Ingredients:
1 tsp. organic cocoa powder
1 tbsp. rolled oats
1 tbsp. milk or half & half cream
1 tbsp. honey

Combine the ingredients and apply the mixture on clean skin and leave on for 15 minutes. Rinse off with tepid water.

RECIPE #10
Bee Pollen & Honey Hydrator and Skin Brightener

This mask is perfect for hydrating and brightening all skin tones.

Ingredients:
1 tbsp. bee pollen
2 tsp. raw honey

Combine bee pollen with raw honey and apply on clean skin. Leave on for 45 minutes. Rinse off with tepid water.

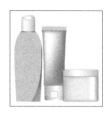

Age-Proofing Tip #21
Age-Defying Skin Care Ingredients

As we reach our 40s, 50s and 60s we begin to notice deeper expression lines, a loss of elasticity and volume, dehydration, hyper-pigmentation or hormonal acne. The good news is we have access to many proven age-proofing products that can help attack free-radicals and aid the skin's ability to repair and renew itself.

As noted on previous pages, twice weekly exfoliation is the key to revealing fresh new cells, reducing fine lines and age spots. To compliment that very important step, I highly recommend integrating topical antioxidants, peptides, epidermal growth factor (EGF) creams, hyaluronic acid (HA), and daily sunscreen. Copper peptides can be used to help firm the skin, address acne breakouts, or broken capillaries.

With so many product choices available to us it can be confusing as when to use these products for maximum efficacy. In addition, many are either overpriced or not very powerful formulations. Below is a guideline of powerful, cost-effective age-proofing skin care products and how to use them.

Once you read through this entire section, you'll gain a clearer understanding of each type of product. Find out more information and where to find the products noted below in the resources guide in **Safe, Effective Face & Body Product Suggestions**.

Epidermal Growth Factor (EGF) – Skin Volumizer

Millions of women over the age of 40 are challenged with loss of volume in the face as well as loss of elasticity. Skin becomes dry, dull, uneven, sunken and dehydrated. By age 50, a woman's skin has lost over 12% elasticity and continues each year that follows, due to hormonal changes. Whether you're aged 40, 60, 80 or more, you can benefit from EGF cream. Scientifically proven ingredient, epidermal growth factor (EGF) has been causing much buzz in the skin care world. It is a scientifically proven, age-defying skin *volumizer* that addresses mature, hormonal skin challenges. It helps regain lost volume in the face and neck, and hydrates mature, dry, thinning, sagging or menopausal skin. Combining EGF with antioxidants and peptides is one of the most powerful skin rejuvenation combinations to date. Read more about the beauty of peptides and antioxidants in upcoming paragraphs.

How does EGF work?

I began recommending EGF creams to my clients in 2011. Originally used to heal diabetic wounds, EGF is made up of blocks of protein that restore the skin's volume and density. The proteins penetrate and bind the cells of the dermis (where collagen forms) and epidermis (surface of the skin) accelerating the formation of thicker, firmer, healthier looking skin with increased volume, elasticity and hydration.

I uncovered two EGF creams that are powerful and cost-effective. One is **De-Aging Solution** with maximum % EGF, antioxidants and super hydrators. The other is **Ultimate Age-Proofing Complex** with maximum % EGF, antioxidants and peptides. Many doctors and skin care spas private label and charge far more for these creams - because they work. I have personally used both creams for about two years and my face looks noticeably fuller. You can see the fullness on the front and back cover photo of this book. Both EGF creams are very popular. In fact, women continue to re-order it over and over again and my European clients usually buy two or three jars at one time. Simply apply EGF cream in the morning, then your sunscreen. Or apply EGF cream before going to bed on face, neck, chest, under and around eyes, and on hands. Find them noted in **Safe, Effective Face & Body Product Suggestions.**

Peptides – Collagen & Moisture Stimulators

Peptides are clinically proven to be more effective than retinoids and vitamin C. I revealed peptides over ten years ago in my first book, and they are often found in many expensive creams. Peptides are like building blocks that restore collagen and moisture in our skin. They reduce inflammation to help rejuvenate aged-looking skin. Peptides can be applied on face, neck, chest, under and around eyes, on hands, stretch marks and cellulite-prone areas. They are safe for all skin types including women who are pregnant and those with mature or sun-damaged skin. Apply peptides morning or evening.

One well-known brand of peptide, called **Matrixyl®**, was used in a French study which proved that peptides can gently exfoliate, smooth, brighten, hydrate and thicken skin. Clinical studies note that Matrixyl® peptides stimulate collagen production *over 360%* and hyaluronic acid production *over 260%*.

Argireline® (AKA Acetyl Hexapeptide-8) is another potent peptide that is proven to reduce the depth of expression lines particularly around the eyes and forehead area by relaxing facial muscles. This topical alternative to Botox® is non-invasive and less costly than injections. Studies reveal that after using Argireline® peptides for just three to six months, wrinkles and furrows are reduced by up to 68% and skin becomes more hydrated. Find Matrixyl® in **Night Perfect**, in **Uplift Serum** and more noted in the peptides section in **Safe, Effective Face & Body Product Suggestions.**

Copper Peptides – For Oily, Mature Skin & Broken Capillaries

Since 1997, copper tripeptide-1 has been referred to as one of the most effective skin regeneration ingredients. Clinical studies have proven that copper peptides increase hydration, promote collagen and elastin production and act as a powerful antioxidant. This skin repairing peptide can help refine superficial scar tissue, even the skin tone and benefits those with acne, age spots, broken capillaries and rosacea. Find copper peptides in **Beyond CP.**

Hyaluronic Acid (HA) – Skin Hydrator

Our bodies naturally produce hyaluronic acid (HA) which hydrates our skin, eyes and joints. But as we age, production slows which can cause dehydrated skin as well as loss of elasticity, sore joints, blurry vision, and more. HA enhances the skin's collagen health providing increased strength and elasticity. It is a natural moisture *magnet* for dry, thirsty skin and can bind up to 1000 times its weight in water. Applying *topical* HA binds moisture to skin resulting in instant hydration. It plumps lines and wrinkles and firms the look of loose skin on the neck and tops of the hands. It even helps plump up lips. See more lip plumping tips in **Age-Proofing Tip #41.** HA is beneficial for those with dry, mature, sun damaged skin with wrinkles or loss of elasticity. Two excellent *topical* HA products are **Uplift Serum** (HA, peptides & antioxidants for face, neck and hands), or **Hyaluronic Acid Hydrating Mist** (HA, antioxidants & natural essential oils for face, neck and body).

Apply either serum <u>under</u> your favorite morning and evening moisturizer. **Hyaluronic Acid Hydrating Mist** can also be sprayed <u>over</u> makeup for a dewy finish that lasts all day. Read more benefits of oral HA supplements in **Age-Proofing Tip #51 - My Favorite Supplements for Women.**

Topical Antioxidants – Nourish & Protect

When applied topically, antioxidants can help repair fine lines, wrinkles, regenerate cell turnaround, fade pigmentation spots, tighten and firm skin and help calm inflammation. They nourish and protect skin from harmful UV rays and free radicals. According to studies performed at *Mount Sinai Hospital in New York*, antioxidants have been clinically proven to maintain healthy collagen and elastin in the skin. Applying a good topical antioxidant should be included in your morning or evening skin care regimen.

Key antioxidants include vitamins A, C and E, Astaxanthin®, Pycnogenol®, resveratrol, CoQ10, alpha lipoic acid, green tea, and DMAE, to name a few of my favorites. Below are highlights of several key topical antioxidants.

Vitamin A (AKA retinoids or retinol) is a skin rebuilding nutrient that speeds cell turnover to help smooth fine lines and wrinkles. Vitamin A is powerful, therefore can cause some redness, dryness or peeling skin. Use it sparingly (once to twice weekly). Vitamin A creams can cause sensitivity to sun so application of daily SPF 15 is required. **NOTE**: Do not use vitamin A products if you are pregnant, nursing or planning to become pregnant.

Vitamin C increases collagen, fights free radicals and reduces inflammation. It comes in various forms such as ascorbyl palmitate (AKA C-Ester) and ascorbic acid (AKA L-ascorbic acid). *Vitamin C-ester* is fat-soluble therefore more stable and gentler than L-ascorbic acid. It is absorbed over time and remains in the skin cells, providing additional UV protection. However, applying daily sunscreen is always best for maximum UV protection. Because vitamin C-ester is stable it does not lose its efficacy.

L-Ascorbic acid is a water-soluble form of vitamin C which tends to be a little irritating to those with sensitive skin. When added to a basic skin cream, ascorbic acid can provide some extra antioxidant power which brightens and evens the skin tone. **NOTE:** Do not add ascorbic acid to a jar of cream as this type of vitamin C loses its efficacy very quickly. For this reason, add the ascorbic acid to *each individual cream application* and apply it immediately on skin.

Vitamin E hydrates, soothes, heals and protects skin from free-radical damage. It is a medicinal moisturizer and is an excellent night time topical lip balm that addresses chapped, cracked lips.

Astaxanthin® is a powerful antioxidant that rehydrates, retexturizes and rejuvenates the skin. It can be applied on all skin types from dry, normal and oily, to those with rosacea, eczema or sensitive skin. Astaxanthin® is derived from micro-algae, 500 times more potent than vitamin E, and 1000 times more effective than beta-carotene or lutein for protecting skin from damaging UV rays. It helps reduce wrinkles and age spots. Find this powerful antioxidant in *Age-Defying Night Crème.* When taken as an oral supplement, it can help reverse the signs of aging both inside and out and even reduces inflammation associated with joint pain. It's truly age-proofing! Read more in **Age-Proofing Tip #47 - Joint Support.**

Pycnogenol®, extracted from pine bark, is 50 times more powerful than vitamin E and 20 times more powerful than vitamin C. Its anti-inflammatory benefits reduce under eye puffiness and redness associated with rosacea and broken capillaries. This is another super antioxidant that contains natural UV protection, fights free-radicals, reduces inflammation, smoothes skin, promotes elasticity, stimulates collagen production and reduces fine lines. Pycnogenol® reduces broken capillaries, redness and fades pigmentation spots. When taken internally as a supplement it helps fade age spots and melasma very effectively. Find it in *Age-Defying Night Crème.*

CoQ10 is one of our most important antioxidants, according to researchers at the *University of Miami.* When applied topically, the enzymes in CoQ10 build up in the skin over time. Applying it consistently can provide skin protecting benefits, reduces the depth of wrinkles and prevents pigmentation spots by protecting the skin from harmful oxidizing UV rays.

Resveratrol is rich in powerful antioxidants that can help sooth and protect skin from free radicals. It is derived from the skin of red grapes is known to fight premature aging. It is found in eye and face creams. Find it in *Eye Perfect.*

Alpha lipoic acid is known as the universal antioxidant because it protects cells from free radical damage. It can deactivate both fat and water soluble free radicals. No other single antioxidant can do this. When combined with vitamin C, alpha lipoic acid becomes even more effective. Find it in *DMAE/Alpha Lipoic/C-Ester Crème,* also known as *Firming Moisturizer.*

Green tea boosts the immune system and keeps skin moist and youthful looking. It replenishes the cells, stimulates collagen, and offers antibacterial properties that help keep blemishes in check. Green tea contains catechins that are known to protect the skin from UV rays. It has been noted in many studies as a topical anti-cancer agent. Green tea is loaded with antioxidants and anti-inflammatory properties so is highly beneficial for all skin types, especially those with oily skin, rosacea or acne. Apply green tea creams on the body with sunscreen on top for even more powerful UV protection. Drinking green tea, taking oral green tea supplements and even bathing in it can help clear blemishes, firm, hydrate and smooth skin. Japanese women have been bathing in green tea for both beautiful skin and relaxation for centuries. Read more about green tea in **Age-Proofing Tip #51 - My Favorite Supplements for Women.**

Gravity-defying **DMAE** can help brighten, tighten and firm skin almost instantly. DMAE contains anti-inflammatory properties that help reduce facial sag, improve skin hydration and tone, and reduce the appearance of lines and wrinkles. It even helps plump up lips. Find it in ***DMAE/Alpha Lipoic/C-Ester Crème,*** also known as ***Firming Moisturizer.***

Transdermal Emu Oil – What is it?

Emu oil is scientifically proven to penetrate the epidermis (surface layers) of the skin. When applied over *any* antioxidant, EGF or peptide-rich product, 'transdermal' emu oil assists the active ingredients of such skin care products to quickly penetrate through the epidermis carrying them deep into the dermis where collagen forms. This can enhance product efficacy. Many plastic surgeons and dermatologists are now advising their patients to apply emu oil after cosmetic procedures to help heal skin and reduce inflammation and scars. Emu oil is rich in omega 3s, 6s and 9s and can help thicken thinning skin without clogging pores. Apply 100% pure emu oil at night over your favorite skin care products for faster skin rejuvenation. See more beauty oils in **Age-Proofing Tip #26 - Beauty Oils**.

Find the products noted above in **Safe, Effective Face & Body Product Suggestions.**

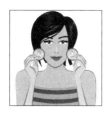

Age-Proofing Tip #22
Universal Skin Care Regimens

Regimen #1 – Mature Normal Skin
(All products noted are free of parabens, phthalates, petroleum, or artificial colors.)

A.M. Regimen

1. Two to three mornings weekly, exfoliate skin with either baking soda or a scrub product such as **Microdermabrasion Scrub**. The other days of the week follow step 2.

2. Cleanse skin with either **Glycolic Facial Cleanser** with Marine Plant Extracts or **DMAE-Alpha Lipoic-C-Ester Cleanser**.

3. Apply **Anti-aging Pycnogenol Toner** to help balance the pH of all skin types. Toner removes any residual cleanser or makeup too.

4. Apply a moisturizer such as EGF cream **Ultimate Age-Proofing Complex** (UAPC) with maximum % EFG, peptides and potent antioxidants to protect and nourish skin, reverse thinning, sagging skin and add more volume to the face. Massage UAPC onto face, around eyes, on temples, crow's feet, jaw line, and neck.

5. Next apply sunscreen such as certified organic **Evenly Radiant Day Crème SPF 15**. This effective non-greasy, hydrating UV cream contains 4.5% zinc oxide and additional UV protecting properties such as vitamin E, vitamin C, green tea, skin brightening Madonna lily, and other skin brightening properties in a natural light citrus scent. It is excellent under all types of makeup too.

6. Lastly, apply makeup. See rejuvenating makeup tips in **Age-Proofing Tip #25 - Look & Feel Younger Makeup Tips**.

P.M. for Mature Normal Skin
(All products noted are free of parabens, phthalates, petroleum, or artificial colors.)

1. After cleansing and toning, apply a peptide-rich serum such as **Night Perfect** or **Uplift Serum** with peptides and antioxidants combined. Or you can choose any antioxidant cream such as **Age-Defying Night Crème** or **Wrinkle Reduction**. You may even alternate one night applying a peptide serum and the next with an antioxidant crème, depending on your budget.

2. For those with mature, dry, deeply wrinkled or sun damaged skin or for faster results with your night time products, massage a drop or two of *emu oil* over any night cream or serum (including peptides, antioxidants or EGF). Emu oil pushes the active ingredients of these potent products deep down to the dermis for faster rejuvenating results. Plus, emu oil can help thicken skin, speed heal incisions and burns and fade scars.

3. Another age-defying combination for mature/dry skin is applying squalane or coconut oil on clean skin one night a week. Or apply either oil under your favorite night time moisturizer. Both oils penetrate and help smooth and hydrate skin. They do not clog pores. Read more about these age-defying oils in **Age-Proofing Tip #26 - Beauty Oils.**

4. Once a week make a home-made rejuvenating mask. Find them noted earlier in **Age-Proofing Tip #19 - Exfoliate Skin, Age-Proofing Tip #20** and in **More Beauty Recipes.**

5. For those with age spots or melasma apply the age spot reducer recipe (below) under any one of the products noted in #1. Or apply **Evenly Radiant Night Crème** three nights a week. It contains several natural skin bleaching ingredients and is organic. To make my age spot recipe **here's what you do:**

Combine 1 tsp. fresh lemon juice with 1 tbsp. witch hazel. Using a cotton swab, spot dab the dark pigments with this mixture. Let dry and then top with the any one of the products noted in #1 or #5.

6. For even faster age-defying results, enhance your skin care regimen with an affordable, rejuvenating LED Red Light Therapy unit. This FDA-approved device repairs damaged collagen for a smoother and wrinkle-free looking complexion. It even helps fade age spots, refines pores and much more. Read more about it in **Age-Proofing Tip #29 - Rejuvenating Gadgets that Really Work.**

7. For those desiring more muscle tone in the face, the exercises noted in **Age-Proofing Tip #28 - Rejuvenating Facial Exercises** are very effective.

8. If your budget allows, consider using a micro-current device twice a month. It addresses muscle tone on the face. You can perform this affordable treatment at home in just 15 minutes. Read more about micro-current in **Age-Proofing Tip #29 - Rejuvenating Gadgets that Really Work.**

Regimen #2 – Dry, Sensitive or Hormonal Skin
(All products noted are free of parabens, phthalates, petroleum, or artificial colors.)

A.M. Regimen

1. Gently cleanse skin with a liquid cleansing exfoliant such as **Glycolic Facial Cleanser** with Marine Plant Extracts. If you like to use a scrub exfoliant, use a little baking soda. NOTE: Do not use scrubs of any kind if you have rosacea. Use a liquid exfoliant such as **Glycolic Facial Cleanser** or **Beyond Clean** (salicylic acid facial cleanser).

2. Next, tone skin with gentle alcohol-free **Anti-Aging Pycnogenol Toner** to remove residual makeup, hydrate and balance the pH of sensitive, dry, oily, or mature skin.

3. If you have sensitive, mature, dry or hormonal skin, EGF cream **De-Aging Solution** is a special *sensitive* skin formulation made with maximum % EGF, nourishing antioxidants and three super hydrators. Gently massage it on face, around eyes, on temples, crow's feet, jaw line, and neck.

4. Apply sunscreen, rain or shine, summer or winter! Try certified organic **Evenly Radiant Day Crème** with SPF 15 zinc oxide protection. It contains skin brightening ingredients such as Madonna lily, licorice root, bearberry and many more healthy ingredients. It's non-greasy, doesn't leave a white film on the skin, and is hydrating and looks great under all types of makeup. It's a lovely sunscreen for everyday wear, winter and summer.

5. Last, apply makeup. See excellent makeup tips for naturally camouflaging spots, acne, blemishes and facial scars in **Age-Proofing Tip #25 - Look & Feel Younger Makeup Tips.**

P.M. Dry, Sensitive or Hormonal Skin
(All products noted are free of parabens, phthalates, petroleum, or artificial colors.)

1 A) At night after cleansing and toning, apply **Age-Defying Night Crème** with potent, moisturizing antioxidants, Astaxanthin® and Pycnogenol®. During winter months or if more moisture is needed, apply emu oil over any night cream or serum (antioxidants, peptides or EGF). Emu oil pushes active ingredients down to the dermis for faster rejuvenating results.

1 B) Another bedtime skin quencher is hyaluronic acid (HA). Apply it on clean face and neck. Two excellent products are **Hyaluronic Hydrating Mist** (with antioxidants) and **Uplift Serum** with (HA, peptides & antioxidants). Spray HA mist over makeup to help set it for the day and provide a dewy, youthful glow.

Regimen #3 – Acne or Blemish-Prone Skin
(All products noted are free of parabens, phthalates, petroleum, or artificial colors.)

A.M. Regimen

For those experiencing teen or hormonal adult acne, below are some highly effective tips that can help clear and prevent breakouts, help fade scars and keep skin looking flawless.

1. Cleanse skin with antioxidant-rich **DMAE Alpha Lipoic C-Ester Cleanser** or **Beyond Clean** (with zinc and salicylic acid).

2. Every morning and evening after cleansing, apply an alcohol-free toner that helps balance the pH of skin such as **Anti-Aging Pycnogenol Toner.** When skin is pH balanced, you will prevent breakouts.

3. For those with oily, mature skin, **Beyond Essential** with Matrixyl ® and copper peptides, antioxidants, and essential minerals is a good choice for day or night.

4. Next, apply sunscreen - rain or shine, summer or winter! Try **Evenly Radiant Day Crème** with SPF 15 zinc oxide protection. It's non-greasy, doesn't leave a white film on the skin, and is hydrating and excellent under all types of makeup. See excellent makeup tips for naturally camouflaging acne and blemishes in **Age-Proofing Tip #25 - Look and Feel Younger Makeup Tips.**

P.M. Regimen for Acne or Blemish-Prone Skin
(All products noted are free of parabens, phthalates, petroleum, or artificial colors.)

1. Be sure to remove makeup before bed. After cleansing and toning skin, apply anti-aging lotion, **Beyond CP,** with copper peptides to help keep blemishes in check, fade spots, broken capillaries and help rejuvenate and firm skin. In the event of a breakout, after cleansing and toning, spot dab blemishes and acne spots with **O24U Hyperoxygenated Gel** using a cotton

swab. Let dry and then apply Beyond CP on top, on the entire face.

2. Exfoliate skin two times a week to avoid clogged or enlarged pores, fade spots, scars and reduce fine lines. Exfoliate using either baking soda (scrub a little onto clean, wet skin), or cost-effective **Microdermabrasion Scrub**. For those with sensitive blemish-prone skin, an alpha hydroxy acid (AHA) cream such as **Evenly Radiant Overnight Peel** is a cost-effective, gentle exfoliant and moisturizing cream all-in-one. It's ideal for those with mature, blemish or acne-prone skin. A third option is applying **024U Hyperoxygenated Gel** as a facial mask once or twice weekly. Whichever method you choose, remember to exfoliate the skin twice a week only.

3. To shrink pores and fade acne or blemish scars, apply the following popular mask twice a week. **Here's what you do:**

Mix 2 tbsp. plain white yogurt with 1 tsp. *fresh* lemon juice. Apply this mask on clean skin and leave on for 30 minutes to help even the tone, fade acne scars, prevent future breakouts, and firm and tighten skin for a face lifting effect. See more masks in **More Beauty Recipes**.

4. Twice a week before bedtime, apply food grade, organic coconut oil on clean skin. It is an effective moisturizer and gentle exfoliator that won't clog pores. Coconut oil contains antibacterial properties, lauric and caprylic, which prevent breakouts. Apply it sparingly.

See products listed in **Safe, Effective Face & Body Product Suggestions.**

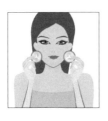

Age-Proofing Tip #23
Winter Wrinkle-Buster Protocol

During winter months our skin requires more moisture. To keep skin nourished, hydrated and protected, apply products that contain effective wrinkle-fighting properties such as peptides, antioxidants, epidermal growth factors (EGF), alpha hydroxy acid (AHA), hyaluronic acid (HA) and beauty oils. See my winter wrinkle-buster protocol below.

A.M. Protocol

1. For mature normal to dry skin, begin by cleansing with a glycolic facial wash such as ***Glycolic Cleanser with Marine Plant Extracts.*** Then apply a pH balancing toner such as ***Anti-Aging Pycnogenol Toner.***

2. Next, apply a face cream or lotion that hydrates and nourishes the skin. The epidermal growth factor creams (EGF) noted below contain skin volumizers, hyaluronic acid (HA) for more hydration, and antioxidants that protect and nourish. Two cost-effective EGF cream choices are ***De-Aging Solution*** (EGF, antioxidants, three super hydrators including HA), and ***Ultimate Age-Proofing Complex*** (EGF, antioxidants, peptides, HA). ***Beyond Essential*** is another excellent hydrating option for those with oily, dry or mature skin. It contains copper peptides to help those with blemish-prone skin as well as hydrating HA and nourishing antioxidants.

3. Next apply an SPF 15 sunscreen such as ***Evenly Radiant Day Crème***. Snow and sun can cause UV ray damage to the skin so it is imperative to apply sunscreen religiously, even during winter. In fact, winter sun reflects off snow and can cause a sun burn!

4. Apply mineral makeup for additional skin protection from UV rays and to camouflage minor flaws, spots or scars.

5. To keep makeup looking dewy, especially during exceptionally dry weather, spray a little hyaluronic acid (HA) mist <u>over</u> makeup. It's amazing how this natural mist sets makeup and hydrates dry, winter skin all day long. I like ***Hyaluronic Hydrating Mist*** (with antioxidants and natural essential oil scent). This is also beneficial for those living in high altitude climates or for those who frequently fly.

P.M. Protocol for Winter Wrinkle-Buster Protocol

1. Each evening after cleansing and toning skin, <u>alternate</u> applications of peptides and antioxidants nightly. For example, three nights a week apply ***Night Perfect*** (peptides in a glycerine base) or ***Uplift Serum*** (peptides in a water base) on face and neck. On alternate evenings apply an antioxidant cream such as ***Age-Defying Night Crème***, loaded with powerful Astaxanthin® & Pycnogenol®. If on a tight budget re-apply ***Ultimate-Age-proofing Complex*** or ***De-Aging Solution*** (noted above in the A.M. Protocol)**.**

2. After applying any one of the products noted in #1, massage a couple drops of ***emu oil*** *on top.* This unique transdermal oil pushes the active ingredients deep into the dermis for faster results. Emu oil does not clog pores and can be used on all skin types. **NOTE:** For those who are vegan or vegetarian, apply squalane oil <u>under</u> your favorite moisturizer for additional hydration. Squalane is derived from olives and will not clog the pores so it is suitable for all skin types.

3. Be sure to exfoliate skin twice a week. See exfoliating choices in **Age-Proofing Tip #19 - Exfoliate Skin** or try either A or B below.

A. Apply ***food grade coconut oil*** on clean skin. It gently exfoliates and hydrates skin. Because it is rich in lauric and caprylic acid, coconut oil keeps blemishes in check too.

B. Apply an ***enzyme peel*** made with organic canned pumpkin. This mask is perfect on all skin types including those with rosacea or sensitive skin. Spas charge about $65 to $85 for an enzyme peel. Make your own pumpkin enzyme peel for under $3. **Here's what to do:**

Combine 2 tbsp. plain pumpkin and add 1 tbsp. honey. Apply on clean skin and leave on for 20 minutes. Rinse the peel off with tepid water.

4. Drink 10-12 glasses of water daily and take omega 3s, 6s, and 9s as well as a daily oral hyaluronic acid (HA) supplement to hydrate skin, joints, eyes and lips from the inside out. Read directions for use on the bottle.

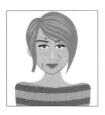

Age-Proofing Tip #24
Blemish and Acne Prevention

I've shared the following effective blemish and acne-prevention tips with many of my clients and customers. These tips can help address some of the reasons for breakouts. **NOTE:** Check with your physician before taking supplements, especially if taking medications or have any diet or health concerns.

*Exposing your face to the sun causes breakouts and enlarged pores! Wear a wide-brimmed visor or hat when spending time outdoors. Apply sunscreen religiously, rain or shine, to bounce harsh UV rays away from skin. Choose sunscreen with inert mineral blockers which will not affect hormones and prevent breakouts. I suggest **Evenly Radiant Day Crème** with SPF 15 zinc oxide protection. It's non-greasy, doesn't leave a white film on the skin, is hydrating and can be worn under all types of makeup. See excellent makeup tips for naturally camouflaging acne and blemishes in **Age-Proofing Tip #25 - Look & Feel Younger Makeup Tips.**

*Avoid eating high carbohydrate / high GI (glycemic index) foods to prevent blood sugar spikes. When blood sugar rises, testosterone production increases which causes *more* oil production AND breakouts. Switch to a low-glycemic diet to keep blood sugar levels balanced. Low-glycemic diets include The Zone, The Mediterranean Diet, The South Beach or Adkins. **TIP:** You can still enjoy a high carbohydrate food from time to time. **Here's what you do:**

Before biting into high carb foods, eat a bite or two of a low glycemic protein-based food such as cheese, meat, or nuts (3-4 almonds, pistachios or walnuts). These types of foods enter the blood stream slowly and help keep blood sugar balanced to prevent breakouts. Then eat the high carb food you wish to enjoy.

*Dandelion root (tea) helps purify the blood and reduces bloating. Drink a cup of dandelion tea to clear and prevent blemish breakouts. Rosemary tea also reduces water retention, blemishes and acne.

*Taking milk thistle supplements can help clear the liver of toxins for a clearer-looking complexion.

*Consuming zinc and soy-rich foods can prevent blemishes and acne. Zinc-rich foods include eggs, liver, seafood, turkey, pork, mushrooms and milk. Soy-rich foods include soy milk (have a soy latte), soy yogurt, soy nuts, soybeans, soy cheese and tofu. You can also apply zinc ointment on blemishes or take an oral zinc supplement to speed acne relief.

*Take omega 3 fatty acids, found in flaxseed oil or capsules to naturally balance hormones and reduce breakouts. Flax is rich in zinc and B vitamins to help combat blemishes. In addition, it's a source of protein and rich in magnesium, potassium and fiber. Take omega 3 fatty acids with meals three times a day. Find them at any health food store. Read the new updates and warning about fish oil supplements in **Age-Proofing Tip #51 - My Favorite Supplements for Women.**

*Chlorella is a super toxin fighter and immune booster which can address acne from the inside out. It clears acne, increases energy and much more. Read many more health and beauty benefits of chlorella in **Age-Proofing Tip #51 - My Favorite Supplements for Women**.

*Tie hair back when exercising or playing sports to keep soiled hands from contaminating hair (that falls by the face). Never touch your face unless hands are freshly washed with soap and water. Avoid resting your face on hands to prevent breakouts.

*Wipe off cell and home phones regularly to remove bacteria that can cause breakouts. Make my hand sanitizer recipe as noted in **Age-Proofing Tip #13.**

*To prevent blemishes, exfoliate skin regularly and wash makeup off before bedtime. Choose cleansers and moisturizers containing salicylic or glycolic acid, alpha hydroxy acid (AHA), soy, sulfur or benzoyl peroxide to help prevent breakouts and clogged pores. See some cost-effective facial cleansers in **Safe, Effective Face & Body Product Suggestions.**

*After cleansing skin be sure to apply an alcohol-free toner to balance the skin's pH. When skin is pH balanced, you'll prevent breakouts. Two excellent paraben-free toners are ***Anti-Aging Pycnogenol Toner*** and ***Vitamin A Glycolic Toner.***

*Exfoliate (slough off skin) regularly to prevent plugged pores and blemishes. Exfoliate using ***Microdermabrasion Scrub*** or baking soda (mechanical scrub). See how to use these products in **Age-Proofing Tip #19 - Exfoliate Skin**. Do not use mechanical scrubs if you have rosacea. Use a liquid or cream exfoliant, also noted in **Age-Proofing Tip #19.**

*Using pressed powder to soak up oil, traps debris and clogs skin, causing more breakouts. Instead, blot oil from face using a hair curler roller paper or grab a piece of toilet seat cover tissue. You can also find oil blotting papers at most beauty supply shops.

*A lightweight makeup primer can help smooth the skin's surface for a flawless-looking makeup finish. It helps fill in recessed acne scars, chicken pox marks and wrinkles on the face. Apply primer over clean, moisturized skin. Then follow with foundation. For primer, Hollywood makeup artists, Debra Coleman and Maria Nguyen recommend **Laura Geller's Spackle®.** It's oil-free and suitable for all skin types. Though it contains some paraben preservatives, as I previously noted, parabens in small amounts are not harmful. However, use it on special occasions. Find it online for about $25. Another budget-friendly choice is **L'Oreal® Studio Effects** for large pores and oily skin. Find it all drug stores nationwide.

*Powder mineral makeup is beneficial for all skin types especially those prone to acne or blemish breakouts. Mineral makeup contains anti-microbial properties that prevent breakouts and provides a natural finish that camouflages acne marks and minor flaws. **Age-Proofing Tip #25 - Look & Feel Younger Makeup Tips.**

See resources for products listed above in **Safe, Effective Face & Body Product Suggestions.**

Topical Blemish Buster Treatments

I've shared the following topical blemish-buster solutions with many of my clients. Apply ONE of the following remedies to blemishes at night. **NOTE:** Do not combine remedies as this may cause irritation.

*Apply **witch hazel** on blemishes using a cotton swab. With the flip side of the swab apply **calamine lotion**. Let dry.

*Apply **milk of magnesia** on blemishes using a cotton swab. Let dry. Magnesium is an anti-bacterial that absorbs oil.

*Apply **saline eye drops** on blemishes using a cotton swab. With the flip side of the swab apply **aloe vera**. Let dry.

*For an open blemish, apply **witch hazel** with a cotton swab. Let dry. Follow with **antibiotic ointment**. Witch hazel disinfects; antibiotic ointment speeds healing and prevents scarring.

*For a large pimple apply **ice** for one minute. Afterward, apply **antibiotic ointment** and leave on overnight.

*When challenged with a 'nest egg' under the skin, consider a high frequency treatment. Aestheticians apply an electrical current on inflamed bumps to kill blemish bacteria. The treatment is painless and offered at most skin care salons on a walk-in basis for around $5. It takes only two to three minutes to zap stubborn blemishes. Within two-three days, the bump is gone.

*An excellent topical formula that addresses acne lesions, blemishes and large 'nest egg' bumps is **O24U Hyperoxygenated Gel**. Apply it on each bump/blemish nightly. Let dry, then apply night moisturizer overtop and leave on overnight. You can even apply **O24U Hyperoxygenated Gel** as a weekly facial mask. It gently peels the skin and fades superficial acne scars.

Back Acne Solutions

*To address back acne apply an AHA (alpha hydroxy acid) cream regularly to help gently exfoliate, hydrate and clear the skin. You may experience some blemishes coming to the surface of the skin for a week or two. Afterward, skin becomes clear with continued twice-weekly applications of AHA. An excellent pH-balanced and cost-effective AHA cream is organic **Evenly Radiant Overnight Peel**.

Another economical back acne remedy is applying a weekly pumpkin mask as noted below. Pumpkin is loaded with enzymes that clear impurities and brighten the skin tone. It also contains vitamin A, beta carotene and other nourishing, skin healing antioxidants. Plain yogurt helps brighten and evens the skin tone. **Here's what you do:**

Combine ½ can of organic plain canned pumpkin with one 8 oz. container of plain yogurt, and stir well. Take a warm shower and pat skin dry. Then apply the pumpkin mask on the back for 30 minutes. Rinse the mask off with tepid water.

*Taking a daily zinc and vitamin D supplement can help keep blemishes in check. Read directions on bottles for dosage. Another excellent supplement for beautiful, clear skin is chlorella. It contains skin-rejuvenating and acne-clearing properties. Read more about chlorella's health and beauty benefits in **Age-Proofing Tip #51- My Favorite Supplements for Women**.

***O24U Hyperoxygenated Gel** is an excellent product for use as a weekly back treatment. Apply it liberally on the back where acne appears. Allow to dry and leave on overnight.

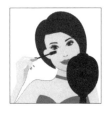

Age-Proofing Tip #25
Look & Feel Younger Makeup Tips

For those with mature skin, you can achieve a youthful-looking complexion by following the makeup application tips below. Your skin is guaranteed to look more fresh and dewy in no time.

1. If prone to eye puffiness in the morning, gently massage a drop of *emu oil* under eyes before bed. Emu oil helps reduce under eye inflammation in about 7 to 10 days. It can even help thicken the eye's delicate, thin skin. Also, avoid drinking beverages about two hours before bedtime and sleep with an extra pillow to prop head up. Sleeping with the head propped, prevents fluids from settling under the eyes.

2. In the morning after cleansing and toning skin, apply an EGF, peptide or antioxidant-rich moisturizer on face, under eyes, on crow's feet and neck. Try *Ultimate Age-Proofing Complex* with EGF, peptides and antioxidants. Another good option is *Beyond Essential* with peptides and antioxidants for normal mature to oily skin types. For those with sensitive, hormonal, mature, or dry skin that needs more volume and hydration, try *De-Aging Solution* with EGF, antioxidants and super hydrators.

3. Next, apply a UVA/UVB sunscreen such as *Evenly Radiant Day Crème* with SPF 15. **TIP:** Allow sunscreen to settle on skin for a moment or two, before applying makeup.

4. Apply illuminating concealer on inner corner of the eyes by the nose and extend to the center under each eye. This prevents emphasis on crow's feet. Try *Boots No. 7® Radiant Glow*; a $13 concealer that works just as well as a department store brand that costs 3 x more! Celebrity makeup artist, Sandra Marshall, introduced this fantastic under eye concealer to me eight years ago and I continue to use it because it offers coverage without creasing. It's perfect for all women over age 35. Hollywood makeup artist, Maria Nyguen, recommends under eye concealer, *Erase Rewind™ by Maybelline®*. She used it for my book cover shot. Both brands offer light-reflective pigments that brighten under the eyes and offer excellent coverage.

5. For those with deep lines, wrinkles or deep acne scars and imperfections, makeup primer can provide a smoother complexion. Apply primer using a foundation brush for a perfectly smooth finish. Makeup primer increases the staying power of

makeup so it's perfect for those special events such as weddings, high school reunions, job interviews and photo shoots.

6. Apply a teeny amount of illuminating liquid foundation just above the cheek bones and blend with a foundation brush. This gives the skin a more lifted and fresh look. Also apply a little illuminating down the center of the nose.

7. Mineral makeup (MM) powder foundation is faster than applying and blending liquid. MM is often sold in dermatology offices because it helps minimize the look of wrinkles, covers blemishes, acne and pigmentation spots or melasma. MM pigments tend to last longer on the skin than most liquid foundations. In addition, MM offers natural UV protection by sitting on top of the skin, refracting UV rays away. Liquid makeup tends to absorb into the skin. However, MM must be applied *sparingly;* otherwise the powdery finish will emphasize lines and wrinkles. In addition, MM is anti-microbial so it is beneficial for those prone to acne or blemish breakouts. Below is the best way to apply MM so it gives skin a youthful-looking glow:

Mineral Makeup Powder Application

STEP 1: Apply ONE THIN coat of mineral makeup onto entire face using a natural Kabuki brush. Buff and blend in the MM using a very light circular touch. This provides a smooth and balanced-looking finish. Afterward, if you still see some blemishes or darker marks and scars, rather than apply another layer of mineral makeup, simply follow step 2 below:

STEP 2: Dip a clean, fine-tipped eyeliner brush into the mineral powder foundation and gently paint over the little dark spots, flaws or blemishes. Then blend the edges to camouflage the marks. This hides spots and scars very effectively and leaves the makeup looking light, fresh and dewy.

8. For a more defined chin or to camouflage a double chin, apply a little bronzer along the jaw line. Be sure to blend it well under the jaw line and down toward the neck using a kabuki brush.

9. For brighter-looking eyes, you'll need a baby pink eye shadow pencil. This is an effective eye-opening tip. Many Hollywood eyebrow specialists charge $23 and up for their baby pink under brow highlighting pencils, but I recently found a great one that is made in Europe, costs half the price of the others and includes a sharpener. **Here's what you do:**

Draw a line of baby pink eye shadow under the eyebrow, and blend it in. This brightens and 'opens' up the eyes. If desired, apply a little of the pink pencil on the inner corners of the eyes too.

10. For more defined brows use a brow pencil or powder. To avoid painted-looking brows, soften the application by brushing brows in an upward direction. See some excellent products and more advice on how to fill in sparse brows in **Age-Proofing Tip #39 - Brighter Youthful-Looking Eyes.**

11. If you like to wear eyeliner, apply it onto the upper eye lid only. This will open and lift the eye. **TIP:** Avoid applying liner below eyes as this causes them to look smaller.

12. To give the whites of the eyes a brighter look, line the inside bottom of each eye with a white eye shadow pencil. I learned this tip from a Hollywood makeup artist when I was a guest on a TV show. For a more dramatic evening look, line the inside of the eyes with a black eye shadow pencil.

13. Curl lashes using an eyelash curler. Apply one coat of mascara to top lashes only. For longer-looking lashes apply a second coat on the *outer third lashes only*. I'm often asked what mascara I use. Since my favorite drug store brand of mascara was discontinued, I was forced to go back to an old department store favorite, **Lancôme® Paris Definicils High Definition Mascara**. Though it's under $30, it's an excellent brand that does not smear and makes lashes look long and thick. It's easy to remove too. See an excellent, cost-effective eyelash growth serum in **Age-Proofing Tip #39 - Brighter Youthful-Looking Eyes.**

14. Apply a healthy, skin hydrating lip balm such as **Chapstick®** (natural formulation) or **Emu Oil Lip Balm**. Then apply organic lip gloss. Glossy, unlined lips appear more plump looking than when lined. And gloss looks more natural and youthful than lipstick. Try a flesh, pink, sheer red or berry-tinted lip gloss and skip the lip liner. And stay away from orange lipstick. It makes teeth look yellow. My current favorite organic lip gloss is **Natural Lips by Aubrey Organics®.** It's made with natural essential oils so it moisturizes lips too. I like pink pearl, strawberry and autumn frost (copper). I also like **Bert's Bee's® Super Shiny Natural Lip Gloss**. See more lip tips in **Age-Proofing Tip #41 - Plumper Youthful-Looking Lips.**

15. Skip finishing powder if aged over 40 because it settles into fine lines which can appear more aging. Instead, blot face

throughout the day using rice blotting papers, hair curler tissue papers or a piece of toilet seat cover.

16. To hydrate skin, spray some **_Hyaluronic Hydrating Mist_** <u>over makeup</u>. It gives the skin a dewy look and sets makeup for the day. This simple tip work wonders!

17. For speedy makeup removal when on the go, I recommend using baby wipes such as natural paraben and phthalate-free **_Seventh Generation_**®.

See the above noted products and where to find them in **Safe, Effective Face & Body Product Suggestions.**

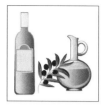

Age-Proofing Tip #26
Beauty Oils

The following oils provide many beauty benefits for all skin types and ages. They can be worn nightly and in some cases applied under your favorite daytime moisturizer or sunscreen. Some of these oils even help reduce scars, restoring skin back to its original skin tone.

Squalane Oil

Squalane Oil, derived from premium olives, is 100% compatible with the natural oils of the face and body. It is similar to skin's natural sebum; therefore it can be used on all skin types without clogging pores. Olive-derived squalane oil hydrates and smoothes the delicate skin on the face, neck, décolletage and around the eyes. It can be used by those with oily, dry, mature, or sensitive skin. Those with rosacea, eczema or psoriasis can safely use this fine, natural oil.

Squalane is often added to costly department store skin care creams. But you can enhance the efficacy of any face cream by applying squalane oil under any nighttime antioxidant or peptide cream. It absorbs quickly to help soften and hydrate even the most delicate skin.

See my facial moisturizer recipe below made with squalane and jojoba oil. Squalane mimics the natural sebum in our skin and can be used on all skin types without causing breakouts. Jojoba oil is rich in plant esters and vitamin E that acts like collagen for plumper-looking skin. It's for all skin types, for battling harsh, winter skin dryness, if living in a dry climate or at a high altitude. I apply my hydrating moisturizer recipe prior to flying to keep skin hydrated. **Here's what you do:**

Combine ½ tsp. squalane oil (derived from olives) with ¼ tsp. jojoba oil and massage on face, around eyes, on neck, chest and on hands prior to bedtime or before a long flight. Flight attendants love my recipe.

Squalane Personal Lubricant

I highly recommend squalane oil as a personal lubricant alternative for all women and men because it's the perfect consistency, isn't sticky, doesn't sting, and is free of parabens, color, fragrance and chemicals. It's a healthy and safe alternative for women experiencing vaginal dryness due to hormonal changes.

NOTE: While researching squalane oil, I discovered that many brands were derived from sharks. I urge you to purchase squalane oil derived from olives. Check with the manufacturer to be certain of the source. As an animal lover myself, I now offer an excellent squalane olive oil brand at a discount price on my website because it is not available at all health food stores.

Find squalane oil in hydrating *De-Aging Solution* with EGF.

Pomegranate Seed Oil

Pomegranate seed oil contains anti-inflammatory properties and high concentrations of fatty acids that nourish and protect dry, mature and sensitive skin. It helps repair wrinkled, sun-damaged skin very quickly. It's an excellent sunburned skin remedy because it acts as a free-radial scavenger to speed heal skin. Find it in skin care creams including *Ultimate Age-Proofing Complex* (EGF cream) and *Beyond Essential*.

Argan Oil

You've likely heard about argan oil for revitalizing hair, but I bet you didn't know that it can be used to rejuvenate and hydrate skin, strengthen brittle nails and fight acne. Argan oil is very rich in essential fatty acids and contains almost twice as much vitamin E as olive oil which it makes it an excellent skin rejuvenator. It does not clog pores and hydrates all skin types. Argan oil helps reduce wrinkles, can relieve eczema, dry scalp, psoriasis and brittle nails. In addition, argan oil's antibacterial plant sterols can prevent acne breakouts. For those with acne, apply the oil under a day or nighttime moisturizer to help regulate oil production. For dry scalp or hair, argan oil is very effective. See how to use it in **Age-Proofing Tip #60 - Fabulous Hair Tips**. **NOTE:** This oil has a natural nutty scent.

Coconut Oil

Versatile coconut oil penetrates the skin very quickly because of its molecular structure. Organic food grade coconut oil is rich in both lauric and caprylic acid making it an ideal natural hydrator and gentle exfoliant for myriad beauty and health concerns including wrinkles, age-spots, acne, yeast infections and sun protection. It strengthens the skin's connective tissue and brightens all skin tones. In addition, the caprylic acid in coconut oil is anti-microbial so it keep blemishes and acne in check. It also addresses yeast and topical fungal infections. Below is a simple topical yeast and fungal fighting recipe. **Here's what you do:**

Poke open 1 vitamin E capsule and combine it with ½ tsp. raw food grade coconut oil. Mix the two oils in the palm of your hand and apply onto fungus or yeast on the skin.

When taken internally, coconut oil's caprylic acid is a natural yeast killer, yet does not affect good bacteria in the intestines. Women living in countries that consume more coconut oil have a lower incidence of yeast infections. Because coconut oil is rich in sun-protecting properties, women who eat coconut oil regularly and apply it topically are known to experience lower rates of skin cancer. During summer months, smooth coconut oil on skin after showering and then apply daily sunscreen on top for extra UV protection.

FACT: Several recent studies are praising the dementia-reversing effects of eating 1 tsp. of raw coconut oil each morning. Reports of those challenged with Parkinson's disease that consumed coconut oil daily, reveal that this remarkable oil can help improve cognitive skills. Choose organic food grade coconut oil. Coconut oil can also be used for cooking. Have a conversation with your doctor if you or a loved one has concerns. **NOTE:** When cooking with coconut oil, go easy. Some individuals report weight gain or loose stools when they eat too much of it. Gradually introduce coconut oil into your diet beginning with 1-2 tbsp. per day.

Rosehip Seed Oil

This skin-healing oil is extracted from seeds grown in Chile's southern Andes. Rosehip seed oil contains powerful retinoids (vitamin A), vitamin E and essential fatty acids which makes it an ideal topical treatment for resurfacing scarred, hyper-pigmented or deeply wrinkled skin. It can soften and smooth sun-damaged, wrinkled skin, crow's feet, and improve the appearance of acne scars, chickenpox, keloids and both fresh surgical and old scars. Rosehip oil can fade red and dark hyper-pigmentation and stretch marks to restore skin to its natural skin tone. It's a natural moisturizer for sensitive, allergic, sun-damaged, post-radiation and burned skin. And is also an excellent treatment for those with dry skin or scalp, eczema, psoriasis, and uneven skin tones. **NOTE:** This oil is highly soothing, though rich in vitamin A and can cause sensitivity to sun exposure. Be sure to apply sunscreen daily when using rosehip seed oil on sun-exposed skin. Find rosehip seed oil in potent facial cream ***Ultimate Age-Proofing Complex*** (EGF cream), ***Beyond Essential***, and ***Beyond CP***.

Emu Oil

Though I noted this in an earlier part of the book, emu oil is one of the best age-proofing oils so I felt it necessary to add it to the **Beauty Oils** section too. Emu oil is non-pore clogging trans-dermal oil that is scientifically proven to penetrate the (epidermis) surface layers of the skin. Applying emu oil over any anti-oxidant, EGF or peptide-rich product assists the active ingredients in penetrating deep down into the dermis (where collagen is stimulated) for even faster rejuvenating results. Many plastic surgeons and dermatologists are now advising their patients to apply emu oil after cosmetic procedures to help heal skin, reduce inflammation and scars and to thicken thinning skin. It's rich in omega 3s, 6s and 9s. Apply emu oil over any of your favorite nighttime serums or creams. The next morning, your skin will look fabulous!

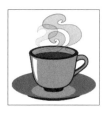

Age-Proofing Tip #27
The Beauty of Coffee

Coffee isn't just a great morning pick-me-up; it's loaded with antioxidants and offers many age-defying properties when applied topically. Drinking coffee uplifts our mood, enhances brain power and is known to help those challenged with depression or dementia. Coffee contains over 400 antioxidants, minerals and phytonutrients including vitamins A1, B1, B2, C, D, E, calcium, magnesium, iron, potassium, zinc, copper, phosphorous and chromium. These properties can protect the brain and body from free radicals. Choose pesticide-free, organic coffee.

A study conducted by the *National Institute of Health* reports that "older adults who drink 2-3 cups of coffee per day (decaf or regular) have a 10% lower risk of premature death than those who abstain."

Save Those Precious Coffee Grounds

When applied topically, the antioxidants in coffee grounds can work wonders on the face, body and hair. Coffee grounds help balance the skin's pH, prevent acne, detoxify, hydrate, firm, smooth wrinkles, reduce cellulite, and more. Be sure to save your precious, used coffee grounds. Store them in a zipper lock sandwich bag and keep them in the freezer until needed.

Coffee grounds gently exfoliate skin and are loaded with skin-rejuvenating antioxidants. In addition, coffee contains polyphenols that balance the pH of all skin types whether normal, oily, acne prone or dry skin. Keep skin hydrated and clear of blemishes with my coffee pH balancer recipe. **Here's what you do:**

First, cleanse face and pat dry. Slightly warm 2 tbsp. used coffee grounds in the microwave for 5 seconds (until warm - not hot). Place a piece of newspaper or paper towel in the sink basin to prevent grounds from going down the drain. While standing over the basin, grab a handful of grounds and gently rub them in a circular motion on face for about 30 seconds. Leave the grounds and antioxidant-rich residue on skin for one minute. Rinse with tepid water. Skin will look rejuvenated and brighter.

TIP: Used coffee grounds keep feral cats out of your garden. Coffee grounds also make excellent mulch for your plants.

See additional recipes in **More Beauty Recipes**.

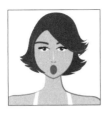

Age-Proofing Tip #28
Rejuvenating Facial Exercises

I can't tell you how many times women email and ask how they can tighten their jowls and jaw line. The following facial exercises REALLY work, and they're easy to perform. And if your budget allows, find more helpful beauty devices in **Age-Proofing Tip #29 - Rejuvenating Gadgets that Really Work.**

Exercise #1 Jowl Tightener

To address a tighter jowl and jaw area, as well as the neck, you will LOVE this highly effective and EASY facial exercise. **Here's what you do:**

Using both pinky fingers, hook one into each side of your mouth. Hold your pinky fingers firmly in place, so they create resistance on either side of the mouth, while saying the word "oh". Repeat 60-120 times. As you resist with your pinky fingers, you'll tighten the muscles of the jowls and up the side of the face. Perform this exercise every other day to firm jowl muscles.

Exercise #2 Jowl & Neck Tightener

This facial exercise addresses both the jowls and neck. **Here's what you do:**

Pull your lips in, wrapping them around the upper and lower teeth. While lips are still in place, smile and hold for 10 seconds. Repeat 12 times. This exercise tightens the jowls and neck muscles.

Exercise #3 Neck Lifter

This neck lifting exercise elongates and strengthens the neck muscles. It helps firm the look of slack neck skin. **Here's what you do:**

To do this exercise, curl your tongue back and hold while you roll your neck back. Hold the neck back for 10 seconds. Repeat 20 times. You may also pivot your head down and up from side to side in a 'U' pattern.

Exercise #4 Double Chin Chopper

To address a double chin, try this easy and effective facial exercise. **Here's what you do:**

While sitting, point your face upward to the ceiling, tilting your head back. Close your mouth and curl the tip of your tongue up to touch the roof of your mouth. While keeping your head in an upward position, open and close your mouth 12 times. Be sure that your curled tongue hits the roof of your mouth each time you close. Then lower your head to normal position and relax for 20 seconds. Repeat two more sets of 12.

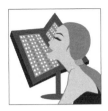

Age-Proofing Tip #29
Rejuvenating Gadgets that Really Work!

"With over 70% of the U.S. population made up of baby boomers, the demand for rejuvenating products is at its highest rate. They are no strangers to seeking non-invasive alternatives to looking and feeling more rejuvenated."

The following age-proofing devices are highly effective, non-invasive treatments that can all be performed in the privacy of your own home. Many beauty professionals and doctors use these actual devices. The results you will achieve are outstanding. In fact, I have posted numerous testimonials on my website from real people and professionals, including doctors and aestheticians who have achieved remarkable results.

LED Red Light Therapy – For Skin Rejuvenation & Pain Management

I revealed the rejuvenating and pain management benefits of LED Red Light Therapy over 10 years ago in my first book. The skin rejuvenation and pain-relieving benefits of LED Red Light Therapy have been clinically proven and documented for decades. And now it is finally being recognized as a proven age-defying device by many famous TV doctors, including Dr. Oz, dermatologist Dr. Eva Shamban, Dr. Ordon and many others.

LED Red Light Therapy is used on the face, neck, hands, arms and body and is scientifically proven to be one of the most non-invasive, economical and effective methods of rejuvenating and plumping wrinkles and fine lines, refining pores, fading age-spots, reducing inflammation, and much more. LED Red Light Therapy can also be used on the body to reduce pain, speed heal wounds, incisions, burns, sprains, pulled muscles and even help broken bones mend faster and better.

How does LED Red Light Therapy work ?

LEDs (Light Emitting Diodes) emit wavelengths of light that enhance the body's ability to repair tissue and damaged cells. This light also stimulates collagen production resulting in plumper, more youthful-looking skin. In just 10 weeks, wrinkles smooth, pores become more refined, age spots fade and much more. The combination of red and infrared LED's and the wavelengths of the lights are the key to its rejuvenating and pain management effects.

For Rejuvenation: The combination of both red and infrared diodes emit specific wavelengths of light that penetrate deep down to the dermis, increasing blood flow to the skin and stimulating the production of collagen to repair damaged cells, refine and smooth wrinkles, plump sagging skin, reduce inflammation and redness, dark spots, enlarged pores and more.

For Pain Management and Reducing Inflammation: The combination of red and infrared diodes of LED Red Light Therapy are also scientifically proven to reduce pain and inflammation in the muscles, back, knees, hands, shoulders, hips and more. LED Red Light Therapy can relieve painful arthritis, fibromyalgia, and aching joints, help speed heal torn muscles, ligaments, sprains, burns, wounds and post-surgical incisions faster and better. Lay the panels on wrists to address carpal tunnel syndrome. To stimulate collagen and reduce the look of cellulite lay the panels on thighs and tummy or strap them around the arms. When applied to the tops of hands, LED Red Light Therapy can relieve painful arthritis and rejuvenate hands by fading age spots.

How to Choose an Effective LED Red Light Therapy Device

An effective LED Red Light Therapy device must combine <u>both red and infrared LEDs</u>. For maximum results, the red LEDs should emit wavelengths that are <u>660 nanometers</u> and the infrared wavelengths, <u>880 nanometers</u>. These are the <u>exact</u> specifications used by NASA when they discovered that LED Red Light Therapy not only rejuvenates, smoothes and plumps wrinkled skin, it even helped heal diabetic wounds very quickly.

The Holy Grail of LEDs

The size of the LED device should also be a factor when choosing a system. This is why I don't recommend handheld units any longer. They are too small, therefore, take far MORE time to complete a treatment and many on the market do not offer the correct wavelengths of light. I suggest a larger 2-panel system which covers the entire face, in far less time. In addition, the high number and combination of 174 red and infrared LED light diodes offer the <u>proven</u> 660-880 nanometer wavelengths - the same specs as used by NASA. This unit can be used at home or in a professional office and it's affordable. In fact, I've set up a huge discount offer on my website so you will pay LESS for a larger unit than you would pay for many handhelds on the market. And the 2-panel system I recommend is FDA-approved and made in the USA. I receive frequent phone calls and emails from countless individuals who report incredible results with the use of this LED. See their testimonials on my website.

I've used a 2-panel LED Red Light Therapy system for countless years - which is one of my key tips to looking younger. Literally thousands of my readers and clients use LED Red Light Therapy for rejuvenating their skin, and calming inflammation or pain. They include doctors, dermatologists, nurses, beauty professionals, spas, aestheticians, the US Army, physical therapists, makeup artists, professional athletes, celebrities, models, TV anchors, producers, directors, moms, baby boomers, and seniors. Even Oprah's O Magazine editor contacted me to send her one.

A Guilt-Free Rejuvenation & Pain Management Device for All

Your entire family, even your pets, can benefit from this remarkable, non-invasive therapy. It is an extremely safe, painless and scientifically proven device that can be used on ANY type or age skin. For decades LED Red Light Therapy has been used by NASA, the US Army and professional athletes to help quickly heal broken bones, torn ligaments, sprains, wounds and more. In addition, veterinarians use non-invasive LED Light Therapy for treating animal injuries and post-surgical healing. See the testimonial of Chris and the amazing unretouched 'before' and 'after' photos of his dog's post-surgical incision. Many women have used the LED to speed mastectomy and breast reduction surgical scars. See many photos of women and men who used the 2-panel system for just 10 weeks to smooth their wrinkles at HollywoodBeautySecrets.com. Be sure to read the testimonials and take advantage of the factory-direct discount I have secured for all of my readers.

As you know, my mission is to uncover the best products on the planet and to offer them at deep discounts to my loyal readers and clients. Find an outstanding deal (almost 30% off), receive *free* S&H in the USA, a 1-year warranty and a 30-day money-back guarantee at my website. **NOTE:** I am not a paid spokesperson for this manufacturer. They process and ship the units factory-direct. I think it's an excellent-quality unit that is priced affordably.

NOTE: Apply the LED Red Light Therapy on clean skin for both rejuvenation and pain management. This will allow the rays to better penetrate the skin. I am often asked if a product can be applied prior to LED use. For years I have recommended using the LED Red Light on clean skin only. However for those with severe sun damage and deeper wrinkles, I recommend ONLY one light-driven product that will not hinder the penetrating rays. It is a thick, gel-like peptide formulation combined with hyaluronic acid (HA) for use specifically with the LED. It is called **Deep Penetrating LED Serum** and can be applied on clean skin prior to use. After the LED treatment, apply your favorite moisturizer over the serum or massage emu oil on top.

Micro-current – for Facial Muscle-toning

Micro-current is a highly effective facial muscle-toning treatment. This device emits low-level electrical currents that alternate positive and negative currents as the unit is moved along the face. In just five to 10 minutes you can treat your face and neck. This proven technology can also improve circulation and lymphatic drainage, and can reduce the appearance of cellulite on the arms, thighs and buttocks.

Using a Micro-current Device

First, cleanse the area you wish to treat. To enhance results apply peptides such as **Night Perfect** or **Uplift Serum**, then the conductivity gel provided with the device. Aloe vera gel can also be used as a substitute natural conductivity gel. Place the probes onto the targeted areas as noted in the instructions provided. As you place the micro-current device on the face, along the jaw line and neck, electrical impulses are delivered via the two probes which rehabilitate and tone the muscles and improve circulation. To get the best results, use a micro-current device daily for about one month. To maintain results use a micro-current twice a month or more. Treatments are available at many spas or purchase your own personal unit.

Enhance Micro-current Rejuvenation Results

For best results be sure to exfoliate skin twice a week with a scrub such as **Microdermabrasion Scrub**. Or twice a week apply AHA cream such **Evenly Radiant Overnight Peel** . Each morning apply either an EGF, peptide or antioxidant-rich moisturizer and follow with sunscreen. See products noted in **Safe, Effective Face & Body Product Suggestions.**

Derma Rollers – for Skin Resurfacing & Stretch Marks

The ***derma roller*** is a device that is manually rolled onto areas such as the face, neck, thighs, stomach or arms. It's an affordable, *semi-invasive* tool that stimulates collagen production and helps retexturize and smooth the look of acne scars and stretch marks. The derma roller can be used to deeply infuse topical serums into skin, enhancing product penetration by a factor of 400%. Apply skin care serums such as hyaluronic acid, antioxidants, or peptides on clean skin first and then use the sterilized derma roller.

Types of Derma Rollers:

The derma roller consists of dozens of tiny needles placed on a small roller. When rolled over a targeted area, the tiny needles create little puncture wounds in the epidermis (top layer of skin). These skin perforations trigger the body to create cell turnover and build up collagen in the area. It's an effective treatment for skin resurfacing.

Some of my clients have commented that their acne and stretch marks have improved immensely after just five derma roller treatments. Compared to costly lasers, they achieved lasting results with virtually no pain or downtime. Derma rollers are far less costly than professional chemical peels and invasive lasers. The treatment can be performed on the face, hands, neck, thighs, tummy, buttocks or arms. Do not use it on or around the eyes. This treatment can be performed by a professional or in the privacy of your own home. I would recommend that you try a professional treatment first to ensure that you learn the proper usage and techniques - especially if planning to use it on the face or neck. Derma roller needles come in three lengths that address different conditions. A quality roller can range in price between $60 and $75 each and many can be found at lower prices on the web. Below are suggestions and length of needles required for each type of challenge or treatment.

0.25 mm derma roller is used on the face, neck and hands for better product penetration, reduction of fine lines, smaller scars and hyper pigmentation problems;

0.5 mm derma roller is more aggressive and can be used on face or body for product penetration, collagen stimulation, hyper pigmentation, smaller scars and hair loss; or

1.0 mm derma roller is medical grade and may cause some bleeding. Use it with <u>caution</u> on deep wrinkles, stretch marks, scars, pigmentation, for collagen stimulation and general skin conditioning on select areas. I do not recommend it for use on the face.

NOTE: Be sure to disinfect the roller prior to use on each area. Do not use a derma roller on moles, on or around eyes, broken or irritated skin, on rosacea or acne breakouts. Consult a dermatologist before using a derma roller.

Facial Flex®Ultra – Cost-effective Facial Muscle Toner

This little gadget has been around for over 20 years! And it is still one of my favorite, cost-effective facial muscle-toning devices to date. No gels or batteries are required. Facial-Flex® Ultra has been used by medical professionals and individuals looking for a natural facelift alternative, with effective results. The muscles that support the face can be strengthened and toned with resistance training. Over time, the Facial Flex® Ultra® provides an effective non-surgical facelift, particularly in the jowl and jaw-line area. It even addresses the muscles on the neck and up the sides of the face!

Clinical studies have proven its efficacy for both therapeutic and aesthetic use, and it has been tested and registered with the FDA. It's a very clever design that is fast and easy to use. You can achieve maximum muscle-toning results in a minimum of time. Using the device just two minutes every other day, result in firmer, stronger facial muscles. The resistance bands for this device are made specifically to generate optimal results and should be changed once a week. Once your facial muscles strengthen, simply switch to a higher resistance weight band or increase the number of reps.

An Affordable Non-Surgical Facelift Treatment

As many of my clients and customers know, I am all about uncovering non-invasive and affordable age-proofing alternatives. I am very excited to introduce a professional face and neck lifting treatment called iEllios II. This impressive technology is very affordable and not only dramatically lifts and firms the facial skin and neck, it requires no down time, laser heat, discomfort, or radio frequency. The cell regenerating currents are developed by the co-inventors of the heart Pacemaker®.

How does it work?

Unlike other skin tightening treatments that stimulate collagen production via use of uncomfortable heat or radio waves that damage cell tissue to rebuild new collagen, iEllios II lifts and firms the skin with zero trauma and far less expense than costly injections and painful face-lift surgery. Though this technology has been in Europe since 2002, it is fairly new to the USA and Canada.

The iEllios II is a medical device which combines science and technology to mimic the body's own electrical micro-currents which trigger protein synthesis and cell regeneration to firm, lift and rejuvenate skin. In addition, it can effectively tighten the sagging jaw line, reshape the facial contours, and can even plump lips!

Unlike fillers and lasers which can cost hundreds to thousands of dollars for just one treatment, the iEllios II costs only $150 or less for a facial treatment. No numbing cream is required. Results can be seen in just two sessions, though usually six sessions are recommended. For those with extremely slack skin, up to 12 sessions may be required. Results can be seen for months afterward. Then a bi-monthly treatment is recommended for maintenance.

Medical aesthetician, Roya Isaacian, at the Brentwood Medical Group & Laser Center is offering a discount off their regular $150/session fee and a complimentary consultation when you call and mention Hollywood Beauty Secrets. Contact at 310-696-0100. In addition, they offer Groupon® rates for laser hair removal and a cutting-edge cellulite and inch loss treatment called Arasis®. Read more about Arasis® in **Age-Proofing Tip #45 - Gorgeous Gams. NOTE:** Prices are subject to change and vary from city to city.

Oxygen Infusion Facial

Another celebrity craze in Hollywood is the intraceuticals oxygen infusion facial. This non-invasive treatment infuses the skin with a series of rejuvenating and skin conditioning serums such as collagen, hyaluronic acid and antioxidants that are administered via an *oxygen* delivery system. The treatment can improve sun-damaged skin and fine lines. Unlike conventional facial treatments, an oxygen infusion facial pushes the nutrients even deeper into the skin, and remarkably, one treatment can last up to 10 days.

The 45-minute treatment includes massage and heat to induce circulation and eliminate toxins, enzymes to help open pores, and customized serums that address several types of skin care challenges from rejuvenation to acne, rosacea or skin dehydration. The result? Skin becomes plumper, more hydrated, youthful-looking, brighter, and dewy. Medical Aesthetician, Aina Kozakov, performs all four customized oxygen infusion facials at Dr. Rubinstein's Dermatology and Laser Centre in Studio City, CA. Though she remained tight-lipped about her celebrity clients, she revealed that some of them come in once a week for the treatment. It's a fairly reasonable treatment that costs around $150 in the Los Angeles area.

Other celebrities who are known to have had this non-invasive facial treatment include Madonna, Victoria Beckham, Eva Longoria, Justin Timberlake, and the lovely Kate Middleton also had a treatment before the royal wedding.

NOTE: Price noted may be subject to change.

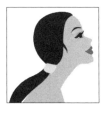

Age-Proofing Tip #30
Botox® on a Budget

There's no getting around it. Those frown lines between the brows and on the forehead can add years to our appearance. Below I've listed a safe supplement, some effective Botox®-like topical products, a home treatment device, and other helpful skin smoothing and wrinkle-plumping suggestions.

*Taking a daily oral hyaluronic acid (HA) supplement can help plump and hydrate the skin from the inside out. This results in younger, lifted, smoother-looking skin. Find HA in all health food stores.

*In addition to taking an oral HA supplement, applying a topical HA product on the surface of the skin can instantly hydrate skin resulting in lifted, softer-looking lines and wrinkles. One of my favorite cost-effective, topical products is **Uplift Serum.** It contains paraben and phthalate-free ingredients including two peptides: 1) Matrixyl® which is scientifically proven to stimulate collagen over 350% and hyaluronic acid (moisture) production over 250%; and 2) Argireline® which softens expression lines. In addition, Uplift Serum contains natural ingredients such as skin firming DMAE, hydrating hyaluronic acid (HA), and powerful antioxidants such as green tea and vitamin C to nourish and protect skin from free radicals. Use Uplift Serum on your face at night or during the day under sunscreen. It even helps smooth the look of loose neck and thigh skin. Many of my clients and customers apply Uplift Serum prior to a high school reunion or special event. It can also be applied *after* using an LED Red Light Therapy device.

*_**Hyaluronic Hydrating Mist**_ is an excellent skin hydrator and plumper that costs under $12. To instantly rehydrate, thirsty, mature skin, apply the mist under your daily moisturizer or spray it <u>over</u> makeup. This sets makeup, resulting in a dewy finish that lasts all day. You may also use the mist as a toner after cleansing. This advanced formula blends the moisture magnetizing properties of hyaluronic acid with antioxidants aloe, green tea, ester-C® and witch hazel in a sparkling water base to promote a radiant, younger looking complexion. The addition of green tea and ester-C® help prevent visible signs of aging. It is naturally scented with phthalate-free essential extract plumeria blossom.

Refill Wrinkle Filler instantly addresses wrinkles on forehead and around eyes. This botox-free, non-injectable wrinkle 'filler' offers an age-defying formulation that can firm the skin tone and smooth wrinkles with continued use. This topical wrinkle filler offers revolutionary age-proofing nanospheres that quickly penetrate into the skin to lift and smooth wrinkles in minutes and lasts for 6-8 hours. Simply cleanse skin, apply on lines and wrinkles around the eyes, nasal labial folds and on forehead. After five minutes, dampen the filler with a little water and apply your favorite day cream on top. The beauty of Refill Wrinkle Filler is that over time with regular use, it continues to smooth wrinkles and build up skin. It contains age-defying active ingredients, including Matrixyl® peptides, DMAE, Retin A®, hyaluronic acid (HA) and vitamins C and E. Peptides are clinically documented to stimulate collagen over 350%, and HA production over 250%, DMAE firms sagging skin, Retin A® and vitamin E and C are topical skin-rejuvenating antioxidants. Additional HA quenches skin and plumps wrinkles. Refill Wrinkle Filler can be used on all skin types including dry, mature, wrinkled, sagging or sun-damaged skin and is free of fragrance or parabens.

LED Red Light Therapy treatments can be performed at home to help dramatically plump, smooth and soften the depth of facial lines and wrinkles. It is one of my key age-proofing tips. Apply the light directly onto clean skin, close eyes and relax for 9-17 minutes. In just weeks, lines and wrinkles become smoother. LED Red Light Therapy is scientifically proven to repair damaged cells and stimulate collagen formation for plumper-looking skin. Read more about LED Red Light Therapy in **Age-Proofing Tip #29 - Rejuvenating Gadgets That Really Work**. It is used by professional and private individuals.

*Exfoliate skin twice a week to banish dry, dead skin cells. In addition, twice weekly exfoliation brings fresh, new cells to the surface of the skin, helps smooth fine lines and wrinkles, and brightens the skin tone.

*Epidermal growth factor (EGF) facial creams help plump, smooth, hydrate and brighten mature skin. EGF helps put more volume back into sinking, aged-looking skin. Two cost-effective choices are *De-Aging Solution* and *Ultimate Age-Proofing Complex.*

Note: Prices noted may be subject to change.

Botox® that Won't Break the Bank

For those who wish to reduce spending on Botox®, a budget-friendly suggestion is injecting one area of face only - between the brows into the glabella muscles. Injecting into this muscle group addresses the frown lines and costs approximately $300. You will save money and achieve subtle rejuvenation that looks natural.

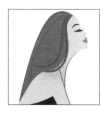

Age-Proofing Tip #31
Neck Lifting Remedies

I'm often asked for tips that address crepe, sagging neck skin. More severe cases are referred to as 'turkey neck.' This occurs due to aging, loss of elasticity and hormonal changes. Below I have noted a few good suggestions for this challenge.

*Each morning, apply some hyaluronic acid serum, such as **Up-lift Serum,** on your neck and top with an EGF (epidermal growth factor) or peptide-rich cream. Then apply sunscreen with SPF 15 on top. An excellent choice is **Evenly Radiant Day Crème.**

*Be sure to exfoliate the neck and décolletage areas two nights a week. However, be sure to choose a cream exfoliant that gently stimulates collagen and brings fresh, new cells to the skin's surface. *Do not* use scrubs on the delicate neck area. An excellent cream exfoliant is cost-effective alpha hydroxy acid (AHA) such as **Evenly Radiant Overnight Peel**. Retinol cream such as prescription Retin-A® is another choice. However, it is a costly cream that can cause dry or red, irritated skin. When using Retin-A® nightly, apply raw, food grade coconut oil or squalane oil on top to help hydrate the skin.

*For the remaining five nights of the week, follow the 2-step regimen below. **Here's what you do:**

STEP 1: Apply an EGF (epidermal growth factor) or peptide-rich cream on neck and chest. Then, follow step 2. If you don't have EGF or peptide products on hand, apply an antioxidant-rich product such as **Age-Defying Night Crème** or DMAE/alpha lipoic/C-Ester Crème. Then follow step 2.

STEP 2: Apply a few drops of emu oil over of any one of the products noted in step 1. As noted in **Age-Proofing Tip #26**, transdermal emu oil pushes active ingredients deep down into the dermis of the skin for faster results.

If you have an **LED Red Light Therapy** unit, use one of the panels on the neck to stimulate collagen and plump skin. **Deep Penetrating LED Serum** can be applied prior to using the LED. This special *light-driven* peptide can speed rejuvenation of the neck and chest when used in conjunction with an LED unit. Afterward, apply emu oil over the serum and leave on overnight.

TIP: When driving, be sure to protect the neck and décolletage from the sun's harsh UV rays that penetrate through the windshield. For this reason keep a long-sleeved shirt in your car. When driving toward the sun, slide the shirt on backwards to block UV rays from reaching neck, chest and arms. Another option is a long scarf. Wrap it around the neck and over the décolletage.

The Instant Neck Lifting Tip that costs Pennies!

This clever little remedy can instantly lift and tighten the look of sagging neck skin. When I share this with friends, they almost fall off their chair in amazement. But it *really* works! It can take five or more years off your age. It's a temporary solution for a special occasion such as a high school reunion, job interview or family photo. **Here's what you do:**

You'll need a hair clip and a 3 ¼" x 1 ½" waterproof bandage. First clip hair up. Then stick one side of the bandage onto one side of the back of the neck - pulling it tightly toward the other side of the neck. Then press on the bandage. This gently lifts and tightens the look of the neck skin. This <u>temporary</u> neck-lifting alternative instantly rejuvenates your look and is far less costly than painful neck-lift surgery. ***NOTE:*** To remove the bandage, lubricate the edges and massage skin with olive, emu or squalane oil. This prevents skin irritation.

*Another neck-lifting option is a product called **Skinnies™ Instant Lifts.** They are skin lifting patches designed to tighten the look of the skin on arms, legs and breasts. Simply custom cut them to size for lifting loose neck skin and follow the directions as noted above. They are a less irritating option than the large waterproof bandage.

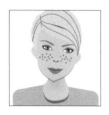

Age-Proofing Tip #32
Fading Spots and Freckles

Pigmentation spots, uneven skin tone, freckles or melasma may be a result of sun exposure, hormone imbalances, contraceptives, pregnancy or childbirth. Check with your doctor before using skin fading products, supplements and tips recommended below:

*Exfoliate skin three nights a week. I recommend using baking soda on wet, clean skin. **NOTE:** Scrub in a gentle, circular motion. Then rinse skin. Another more powerful scrubbing option is **Microdermabrasion Scrub**. It's a phthalate and paraben-free thick scrubbing paste consisting of volcanic ash, dead sea salts and other natural ingredients. Many report that after just three uses, it's just as effective as having had a professional spa treatment. Read more methods of exfoliation in **Age-Proofing Tip #19 - Exfoliate Skin**.

*After exfoliating, rinse skin and pat dry. Then apply a peptide-rich serum or lotion such as **Uplift Serum, Night Perfect** or **Beyond Essential**. Peptides stimulate collagen, brighten and even the skin tone as well as hydrate mature skin. Read more about peptides in **Age-Proofing Tip #21 - Age-Defying Skin Care Ingredients**.

*Sun causes pigmentation spots on the face. Be sure to apply sunscreen, rain or shine, to protect skin from the sun's harmful UV rays. Choose products that contain zinc oxide and titanium dioxide. They are inert blockers that won't disrupt hormones because they remain on the surface of the skin. These blockers refract UV rays *away* from the skin. An excellent moisturizer and sunscreen-in-one is **Evenly Radiant Day Crème** SPF 15 with UVA/UVB protection and skin brighteners that help fade spots. It looks great under makeup (powder mineral or liquid foundation) and is hydrating without leaving a white or greasy film on the skin. It contains 4.5% zinc oxide and additional UV protecting properties and antioxidants including green tea, vitamin C, E, and skin brightening Madonna lily, licorice root, bearberry, and niacinamide in a light, natural citrus scent.

*If planning to be outdoors for over two hours, be sure to increase sun protection to 30 SPF and apply sunscreen every two hours. I like **Aubrey Organics® Natural Sun 30+, and Neutrogena® Pure & Free Liquid Daily Sun Block.** For added UV protection, I suggest wearing a wide-brimmed sun visor or hat to provide a physical block from the sun's harsh rays.

*At bed time, apply a skin care lotion, cream, or mask that contains ingredients such as Pycnogenol®, vitamin c-ester-, alpha hydroxy acid (AHA), retinol (vitamin A), peptides, soy, pumpkin or papaya. Other skin fading ingredients to look for on labels include Madonna lily, licorice root, milk thistle, bearberry, niacinamide, ginseng, alpha lipoic acid, kojic acid, lactic acid, glycolic acid, orange or lemon juice. Below are more details about these powerful, skin-brightening ingredients:

-Taking a supplement such as **Pycnogenol**® can address spots and melasma from the inside out. One study revealed that Pycnogenol® significantly lightened over-pigmented areas like sun spots and melasma. Women in the study took 75 mg Pycnogenol® supplements daily for one month, resulting in a significant reduction in pigmentation. Those challenged with melasma may find this supplement highly beneficial. It's anti-aging too. Find pycnogenol® supplements at most health food stores.

-Topical **vitamin c-ester** serum is a fat soluble, powerful antioxidant that protects skin from UV damage, fades pigmented spots and contains anti-inflammatory agents to help prevent and repair fine lines and wrinkles. It builds up within the skin's cells for continued protection from free radicals.

-**Alpha lipoic acid** is found in many types of antioxidant creams. It gently exfoliates the skin, unclogs pores and can help fade pigmentation spots over time. You'll notice skin tones evening out in just two to three months.

-**Retinol** (vitamin A) is a prescription skin exfoliant that can help fade pigmentation spots and reduce lines and wrinkles. It can be irritating to those with sensitive skin and not recommended during pregnancy. Apply sunscreen daily if using retinol as it causes sensitivity to the sun's UV rays.

-**Peptides** can help gently brighten and even skin tone. Peptides have been proven to be gentler, yet more effective than retinol. In addition, peptides stimulate collagen and hyaluronic acid production in skin and are safe for use during pregnancy.

-**Lactic** and **glycolic acids** are derived from milk or plants and are found in many creams and cleansers. They can help brighten skin and fade pigmented areas. **Glycolic Cleanser with Marine Plant Extracts** is popular, healthy and cost-effective.

-Madonna lily, licorice root, milk thistle, bearberry, niacina-mide, ginseng, alpha lipoic acid, kojic acid, lactic acid, glycolic acid, orange and lemon juice are natural, skin-bleaching agents found in creams and cleansers. An excellent skin brightener that contains several of the above-noted ingredients is **Evenly Radiant Night Crème.**

*Wear a shirt with long sleeves, a cotton scarf and gloves to protect neck, chest, arms and hands from UV rays. Also, exercise after 5:00 p.m. to prevent pigmentation damage.

*LED Red Light Therapy is an affordable, non-invasive and effective treatment that can help diminish pigmentation spots. No down time or pain is involved. Many celebrities are opting for LED Red Light Therapy because it can repair and prevent wrinkles by stimulating collagen production.

*Mineral makeup (MM) can naturally camouflage pigmentation spots. The trick is to apply it sparingly for a natural finish. Apply MM using a gentle, light-handed buffing motion. Then touch up darker spots using a fine-tipped, clean eyeliner brush. Lightly paint over little flaws and scars for a dewy, fresh look.

*Coconut oil contains natural hydrating, skin brightening and gentle exfoliating properties. **Here's what you do:**

After cleansing and toning skin, apply coconut oil three nights weekly. TIP: Apply it sparingly for better absorption. Read more about coconut oil in **Age-Proofing Tip #26 - Beauty Oils.**

*A Los Angeles physician shared this skin-lightening recipe with me. It's made with **multani mati**, an herbal clay powder available at most Indian food stores. **Here's what you do:**

Combine two parts multani mati with one part emu or squalane oil and apply on clean skin. Leave on for 30 minutes and then rinse off with tepid water. You'll be left with a brighter-looking complexion.

*Turmeric is an antioxidant-rich spice that offers skin lightening properties. Turmeric has long been used as a powerful anti-inflammatory in both Chinese and Indian medicine. In addition, turmeric offers anti-inflammatory benefits which can help calm the redness associated with rosacea. See my skin brightening mask made with turmeric in **More Beauty Recipes**.

See products noted above in **Safe, Effective Face & Body Product Suggestions**.

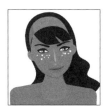

Age-Proofing Tip #33
Banishing Milia

Sun damage, aging and lack of exfoliation are common causes of milia. They appear as tiny white bumps that look similar to whiteheads. However milia are a result of dead skin cells that become trapped in the pores, and are not caused by sunscreen or product buildup, as many assume. Milia can be reduced and prevented with regular exfoliation. As mentioned on earlier pages, exfoliating the skin two to three times a week stimulates collagen production and brings new, fresh cells to the surface. Preventing milia is another reason to exfoliate skin two to three times weekly. See some helpful exfoliating choices below.

*Cost-effective scrubbing paste **Microdermabrasion Scrub** is made with volcanic sand and other natural ingredients. It is a healthy, powerful scrub that can remove and prevent milia. Another option is using an exfoliating cream such as alpha hydroxy acid (AHA) cream. Also facial cleansers that contain glycolic or salicylic acid are good choices. Some excellent products include **Evenly Radiant Overnight Peel** (AHA cream), **Beyond Clean** (salicylic acid cleanser) or **Glycolic Cleanser with Marine plant extracts.**

*In extreme cases seek a mild chemical peel (salicylic acid) or a professional microdermabrasion treatment.

*Apply **retinol** (AKA retinoids or Retin-A®) twice weekly. It is a prescription cream that speeds cell turnover. Once milia are smoothed away, use retinol once a week only to prevent thinning the skin.

*As a last resort, milia can be extracted using a comedone extractor, which 'digs' out the bumps. However, this procedure must be performed by a dermatologist. Some Russian and Israeli-trained aestheticians are highly skilled in milia extraction as well. But be aware that removal requires lancing the skin and may result in a small hole or scar. To speed heal skin and prevent scarring, I suggest using an **LED Red Light Therapy** unit after the treatment for a week or two. If you do not have an LED Red Light unit, other options are nightly applications of vitamin E or an anti-biotic ointment such as poly or Neosporin®. Honey is another excellent natural anti-microbial and antibiotic skin healer that can be applied after milia extraction.

See the above noted products and where to find them in **Safe, Effective Face & Body Product Suggestions.**

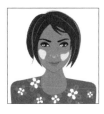

Age-Proofing Tip #34
Camouflaging Vitiligo

Vitiligo is a skin condition that is caused when the immune cells attack the natural pigmentation (melanin) in the skin causing white patches to appear on the face, hands and body. Vitiligo affects approximately one in 100 individuals in North America. It appears in varying degrees in many skins types and until now, has been difficult to camouflage. You may recall that Michael Jackson was challenged with this autoimmune condition. There is no cure for vitiligo; however, there are some measures one can take to make this condition less noticeable.

*Avoid sun exposure as UV rays darken the surrounding skin of the white patches causing them to look more pronounced. During summer months, wear lightweight cotton clothes to camouflage arms and legs.

*Self-tanning moisturizer **Tan Toner** can help camouflage the look of vitiligo and patchy skin. It is paraben and phthalate-free (synthetic fragrance) and gradually darkens whitened areas on the skin without disrupting hormones. Its key properties include a melanin producing peptide, stem cells from grapes, a skin-firming anti-aging peptide and other powerful antioxidants to help repair skin damage. This self-tanner is a moisturizing age-proofing product too. Independent studies revealed a 20% increase in elasticity and firmness after just 28 days of use. Unlike other commercial self-tanners, Tan Toner contains a very mild and pleasant scent made with natural extracts. The natural scent dissipates quickly too. This new product provides a healthy-looking tone, without the orange pigments that stain or sweat off.

How to Camouflage Vitiligo

To camouflage vitiligo, first apply **Tan Toner** onto the lightened patches to restore color back to normal skin tone. Once the skin looks even, apply the self-tanner over the entire area every 5-7 days to maintain color. If darker, more tanned looking skin is desired, wait 24 hours between applications until you reach the desired tone.

See the above noted products and where to find them in **Safe, Effective Face & Body Product Suggestions.**

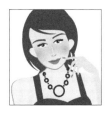

Age-Proofing Tip #35
Relieving Rosacea

Those challenged with rosacea may greatly benefit from the following remedies. However, consult with a dermatologist first.

*Cleanse skin with liquid 2% salicylic acid cleanser or a glycolic acid based cleanser. Both cleansing products gently exfoliate skin while reducing inflammation and redness without irritating skin. Both **Beyond Clean** cleanser (salicylic acid and zinc) and **Glycolic Facial Cleanser with Marine Plant Extracts** are free of phthalates, synthetic color, petroleum and parabens.

*The following antioxidants creams and oils are excellent choices for those with rosacea and sensitive skin. Topical Pycnogenal® cream or gel can benefit the capillary system and help reduce redness and inflammation associated with rosacea. Find **Pycnogenol® Gel** at select health food stores. It is also present in **Age-Defying Night Crème. Sea Buckthorn Oil** is known to calm dry, red and inflamed skin, especially during the winter months. The oil is rich in quercitin, an antioxidant that calms and reduces redness and irritated dry skin. **Squalane Oil** derived from olives mimics the skin's sebum and hydrates sensitive skin conditions such as rosacea.

*Antioxidant-rich **green tea** offers anti-microbial and anti-inflammatory properties that calm redness and blemishes associated with rosacea. **Here's what you do:**

Place two green tea bags in warm water to release the healing tannins. Then dab tea bags onto red areas for five minutes. Or apply a simple green tea moisturizer.

***Olive Gold 03** suspends super oxygen molecules in ozonated olive oil, allowing deep penetration into skin. It contains antibacterial, antifungal and antiviral properties that can help relieve rosacea.

***Propolis** is made by honeybees and used as a form of bee 'glue' to construct and protect their hives. Propolis is derived from plants and botanical sources and is rich in antioxidants such as beta-carotene, vitamin C and E to help calm the redness and inflammation associated with rosacea, eczema, or psoriasis. It can be taken orally or applied topically.

*Scrubbing, rubbing, using abrasive exfoliants or wash cloths exacerbates rosacea. Apply an alpha hydroxy acid (AHA)cream for gentle exfoliation, hydrating and brightening skin.

*__Vitamin B-12 injections__ and applying __B-12 creams__ have been known to help remedy rosacea. A compounding pharmacy should be able to make a B-12 cream for you. Be sure to mention that you wish the base emollient be organic or free of phthalates and parabens.

*Avoid saunas, sun exposure, hot tubs, cold winds, exfoliants, stress, spicy foods, hot beverages and smoking as they can trigger an outbreak of rosacea.

*Eating cheese can trigger histamine production that causes redness. Other foods to avoid include sour cream, yogurt, chocolate, soy sauce, vinegar, navy beans, lima beans, pea pods, spinach, eggplant, tomatoes, bananas, citrus fruits, raisins, plums, figs and liver.

*Recommended foods include antioxidant-rich vegetables such as broccoli, artichokes, asparagus, green beans, leafy lettuces and fruits such as blueberries, raspberries, strawberries, blackberries, peaches, plums and cantaloupe.

*Avoid alcohol (red wine, vodka, gin, beer, champagne and bourbon) hot coffee, tea, cider, and chocolate.

*Avoid cosmetics and products containing synthetic fragrance (phthalates), synthetic color, alcohol, peppermint, witch hazel, menthol, retinoids and facial scrubs.

*Taking zinc and vitamin A supplements daily can help minimize rosacea.

*Mineral makeup can help camouflage redness associated with rosacea.

*Turmeric is an antioxidant-rich spice that has long been used as a powerful anti-inflammatory in both Chinese and Indian medicine. It can help calm the redness associated with rosacea. See my skin brightening mask made with turmeric in **More Beauty Recipes.**

*LED Red Light Therapy can help calm and reduce the red flush and inflammation associated with rosacea. In addition, LED Red Light Therapy helps smooth wrinkles, refines pores, and fades pigmentation spots and much more. Read more about

LED Red Light Therapy page in **Age-Proofing Tip #29 - Rejuvenating Gadgets that Really Work.**

*A series of IPL photo facials can help reduce rosacea and pigmentation problems via broad spectrum rays that reduce redness. However, they can be costly at about $250 to $500 a session. Usually five to six sessions are required. Pulse dye lasers also address broken blood vessels.

*Visit www.rosacea.org for more information.

Find products noted in this section in **Safe, Effective Face & Body Product Suggestions.**

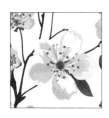

Age-Proofing Tip #36
Relieving Eczema

This skin disorder causes inflamed, red areas or dry patches on the skin. Wind, extreme temperatures, hot or cold water, anxiety and stress may trigger an outbreak of eczema. Consult a dermatologist. Eczema cannot be cured. However, there are many steps one can take to keep this condition in check.

***Borage** and **flaxseed oil supplements** are rich in essential fatty acids (EFA) and clinically proven to help ease dry skin such as eczema. Take a combination borage-flaxseed oil supplement with meals three times a day. Read more health facts and hormone-balancing effects of omega-3 flaxseed oil supplements in **Age-Proofing Tip #51 - My Favorite Supplements for Women.**

***Dandelion tea** is a powerful blood purifier that can calm dry skin conditions such as eczema and psoriasis. Drink dandelion root tea daily. Other good teas are ginger or chamomile. Add honey to any one of these teas for additional calming and natural antibiotic properties.

*Many studies note that stress can trigger an outbreak of eczema. Try **Rescue Remedy®** oral spray made with wild flowers and plants for natural calming. Supplement **5-HTP** is another non-habit-forming, drug free day or evening de-stresser. Read more tips in **Age-Proofing Tip #9 - Brain Boosters & Good Mood Foods.**

***Propolis** is made by honeybees to protect their hives. This sticky glue-like substance is derived from plants and botanical sources and is rich in antioxidants such as beta-carotene, vitamin C and E to help calm the redness and inflammation associated with eczema, psoriasis or rosacea. Propolis can rapidly heal cracked, dry patches, wounds and burns. **NOTE:** Do not use propolis if allergic to bees, etc.

***Bee pollen** and **honey** are known to help eczema. The Chinese tonic recipe below is effective. **NOTE:** Do not use this recipe if allergic to bees, etc. **Here's what you do:**

Combine 2 tbsp. bee pollen, 2 tbsp. raw honey, 1 tbsp. ginseng extract to a cup of hot water. Stir and drink each morning.

112

The following nightly topical treatment is effective too. **Here's what you do:**

Combine 1 tsp. bee pollen with 2 tsp. emu oil and apply onto patches. Cover with gauze. Leave on overnight.

__Milk thistle__ is an oral supplement that can help relieve eczema, detoxify the liver and can balance hormones. Take it seasonally. Check with your doctor before taking supplements. Another benefit I recently read about milk thistle is that it may play a part in delaying tumor growth.

*Eliminate or reduce dairy. Soy, goat or sheep cheeses are preferable substitutes. Shellfish, sugar, yeast, strawberries and pineapple may exacerbate eczema.

*Foods such as peas, snow peas, split pea soup and ginger soup are good choices for calming eczema. In addition, foods rich in B6 are beneficial. They include bell peppers, spinach and summer squash.

*Fatty acids in oatmeal moisturize dry skin and reduce inflammation. Oatmeal lotions and/or oatmeal baths offer immediate relief. **Here's what to do:**

Pour 1 cup oatmeal into a tepid bath and soak for 20 minutes. Do not rinse skin. Simply pat skin dry.

*Another excellent remedy for eczema is a chamomile bath: **Here's what to do:**

Steep 10 chamomile tea bags in 3 cups boiling water. Remove tea bags, and pour chamomile tea into tepid tub water. Tannins in chamomile can help relieve inflammation and dry, itchy skin. Don't rinse skin. Simply pad skin dry.

*New studies report that taking probiotics can help alleviate eczema. Read more benefits of probiotics in **Age-Proofing Tip #51 - My Favorite Supplements for Women.**

*A study performed in Europe revealed that applying a *__B12 cream__* can also help relieve eczema. Visit your local compounding pharmacy to make a formulation using 0.07% strength B12. Request a cream base that is free of parabens and phthalates.

__Rosehip seed oil__ is a natural moisturizer for sensitive, sun-damaged, post-radiation and burned skin. And it's an excellent treatment for those with dry skin, eczema, psoriasis, and uneven skin tones. **NOTE:** This oil is highly soothing, though rich in vitamin A and E. It can cause sensitivity to light so apply sunscreen.

*Both **vitamin E** and **vitamin B3** are known topical remedies that relieve the epidermis (surface skin layers) of dryness. Vitamin E is a skin hydrator and smoother while niacinamide in vitamin B3 calms skin.

*Using a 2% salicylic acid cleanser gently exfoliates (sloughs off) dry skin without irritation. Try paraben, fragrance, and dye-free **Beyond Clean Cleanser** with salicylic acid and zinc.

*Witch hazel can also help calm eczema. Use a cotton ball to apply it.

*Another excellent remedy for dry skin issues is applying topical liquid organic **echinacea** directly onto dry patches as well as taking it as an oral tincture 4-5 times a day. Echinacea is a well known-immune booster.

***Olive Gold 03** suspends super oxygen molecules in ozonated olive oil allowing deep penetration into skin. It offers antibacterial, antifungal and antiviral properties that can help relieve eczema and has myriad other topical skin applications.

*Temporarily clear dry patches with hydrocortisone cream. Reduce use after seven days.

*Super green marine algae chlorella is an excellent skin rejuvenator that offers many head-to-toe benefits including those challenged with dry skin issues such as eczema. Read more about it in **Age-Proofing Tip #51 - My Favorite Supplements for Women.**

See products noted above in **Safe, Effective Face & Body Product Suggestions**.

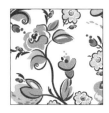

Age-Proofing Tip #37
Relieving Psoriasis

This disorder causes inflammation, scaling, and flaky, itchy patches on skin. Consult a dermatologist.

*Archives of Dermatology reports that fungus living in the lesions on the skin may cause psoriasis. Sugar stimulates production of fungus. Avoid sugar, high-glycemic foods such as candy, soft drinks, ice cream, cereal, pastries, pudding, bread, rice, pasta, rolls, green peas, corn, beets, potatoes and grains. Choose low-glycemic fruits such as blueberries, cantaloupe, raspberries, strawberries and kiwi. Choose vegetables such as dark and leafy greens, celery, red and green peppers, brussel sprouts, broccoli, cabbage, radishes, tomatoes and turnips.

*Wash with 2% salicylic acid cleanser to reduce flaky, dry patches. Try paraben and phthalate-free ***Beyond Clean Cleanser***.

****Oil of oregano's*** anti-fungal and antibacterial properties relieve lesions, dryness, inflammation, itching, swelling and soreness. Apply oil on each area twice daily. In addition, taking oil of oregano orally can help calm this challenge. Place three to four drops of oil of oregano into a gelatin capsule and take one capsule daily with meals.

*Another excellent remedy for dry skin issues is applying topical liquid organic **echinacea** directly onto dry patches three times a day. In addition, taking echinacea as an oral tincture 4-5 times a day can help calm psoriasis and eczema. Echinacea is a well-known immune booster.

****Sea buckthorn oil*** is known to calm dry, red and inflamed skin, especially during the winter months. The oil is rich in quercitin, an antioxidant that calms and reduces redness and irritated dry skin.

****Coconut oil*** contains caprylic acid which can calm inflammation, and gently exfoliates and hydrates skin.

****Rosehip seed oil*** is a natural moisturizer for sensitive, allergic, sun-damaged, post-radiation and burned skin. And it's an excellent treatment for those with dry skin challenges such as psoriasis or eczema. **NOTE:** This oil is rich in vitamin A and E. Though rosehip seed oil is highly soothing, it can cause sensitivity to light so apply sunscreen daily.

*A study performed in Europe revealed that applying a **B12 cream** can help relieve dry skin challenges such as psoriasis and eczema. Visit your local compounding pharmacy to make a formulation using 0.07% strength B12. Request a cream base that is free of parabens and phthalates.

*For psoriasis patches on scalp, massage pure **argan oil** into scalp and throughout hair and leave on overnight. Then shampoo hair as usual in the morning.

*A daily application of **vitamin c-ester** reduces redness and scaling associated with psoriasis. Improvements can be seen within three to four months use.

*Taking a **flax-primrose** and **borage oil** combination supplement can help relieve psoriasis.

Milk thistle can help relieve psoriasis as well as detoxify the liver and balance hormones. Take it seasonally. Check with your doctor before taking supplements.

See the above noted products and where to find them in **Safe, Effective Face & Body Product Suggestions.**

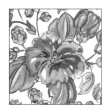

Age-Proofing Tip #38
Combating Keratosis Pilaris
(Chicken Bump Skin)

Keratosis Pilaris, also known as chicken bump skin, is hereditary and affects 50% of the world's population. Keratosis Pilaris may not be curable because it is genetically predetermined though it can be controlled. These sandpaper-like brownish-red bumps are most frequently scattered along the upper arms, thighs, back or buttocks and can be embarrassing for some. Keratin scales prevent hair from reaching the surface and cause the raised bumps to develop beneath inflamed hair follicles. Because the normal shedding of old skin cells does not occur regularly, the skin becomes rough, bumpy and uneven in texture. These bumps can be unsightly. However, regular exfoliation can help.

Below are some effective protocols:

1) **Retin A** can be applied daily for two to three weeks to initiate powerful exfoliation. To maintain skin smoothness, twice daily applications of lactic acid, alpha hydroxyl acid (AHA), or vitamin C cream are required.

2) For more severe cases, consider getting a series of professional microdermabrasion treatments which can speed results. Then maintain results with twice-daily applications of any one of the exfoliating lotions noted in #1. Another less costly, yet highly effective product is topical **Microdermabrasion Scrub** made with volcanic sand and dead sea salts. It is highly abrasive, therefore very effective for this condition. It is free of parabens, synthetic fragrances (phthalates), petroleum and color.

3) A light chemical peel can help initiate exfoliation. Follow with twice-daily topical exfoliating creams and a twice-weekly scrub as noted in #2 to keep chicken bump skin in check. See your dermatologist for a professional chemical peel.

4) An excellent daily after-shower hydrator and gentle exfoliator is **Skinlasting Super Hydrator**. It is rich in skin-exfoliating lactic acid and free of parabens, synthetic fragrances (phthalates), petroleum and color.

See the above noted products in **Safe, Effective Face & Body Product Suggestions.**

Age-Proofing Tip #39
Brighter, Youthful-Looking Eyes

"The eyes are the windows of the soul."
– Leonardo DaVinci

The following tips can help protect and rejuvenate the eyes, prevent cataracts, and more.

Protect eyes by consuming omega-3 fatty acids including fresh fish, flaxseed and evening primrose oil, walnuts and antioxidant-rich red, orange and green fruits and vegetables including avocados, leafy greens, kale, broccoli, spinach, tomatoes, red and orange bell peppers, papayas, apples, and oranges to name a few.

Though the property lutein, found in tomatoes, is known to help eyes, recent studies reveal that the antioxidant **Astaxanthin®** is an even more powerful supplement for eye health and it may play a role in preventing blindness. Because it can enter the retinal barrier of the eyes, it can reduce risk of glaucoma, macular degeneration and cataracts. In addition, it's a rejuvenating antioxidant for skin, reduces inflammation and joint pain when taken orally. Astaxanthin® is 500 times stronger than vitamin C. It is naturally orange in color and found in foods such as lobster, salmon and shrimp. Read more about Astaxanthin® in **Age-Proofing Tip #47 - Joint Care.**

Hyaluronic acid (HA) supplements can be highly beneficial to those with dry eyes or deteriorating sight. As we age, our bodies produce less HA which is one of the reasons eyesight declines and many individuals require reading glasses by age 40. Taking HA in supplement form is known to improve sight, provide pain relief, cushion joints and keep skin and lips hydrated, plump and more youthful-looking.

*Wear sunglasses when outdoors. Several studies have proven that protecting eyes from harmful UV and UVB rays can prevent the onset of cataracts. Choose **polarized sunglasses** as they are known to provide extra UV protection. Also avoid tanning beds which also emit harmful UV rays.

*To promote eyelash growth, nourish and condition lashes, apply **argan oil.** It is 100% natural and derived from a nut grown in Morocco. After cleansing, massage a drop of argan oil onto lashes. Gently massage a little oil under eyes for moisture too. Leave on overnight.

RapidLash® Eyelash & Eyebrow Enhancing Serum is a super effective and affordable nightly treatment that works wonders on eyelashes and brows! It's a non-prescription strength formulation with powerful peptides that protect against breakage, vitamins including panthenol and minerals to nourish hair, and protein for luster. It's also free of parabens, phthalates or fragrance. I gave it to three women to try. Two of the three gals used it religiously and they both achieved longer lashes. I also put RapidLash® to the test. Though Mom and Dad blessed me with long lashes, I was curious to see if I would achieve a noticeable result. Within six weeks, my eyelashes were remarkably longer. In fact, some of them grew to ½" in length! Amazing stuff!

*Thicker brows can rejuvenate your look. If you've got thin, over-tweezed brows, there is hope. Eyelash enhancing serums can also help growth of sparse brows. I tried a couple different brands on each eyebrow and I experienced faster results with cost-effective *RapidLash® Eyelash & Eyebrow Enhancing Serum.* In fact, it was half the price of the other brand I tested. In just seven weeks of daily and nightly use, my brows were much fuller. I've recommended it to many women.

*To instantly fill in eyebrow gaps, *Brow Wiz®* brow pencil by Anastasia mimics the look of real brow hair. It's an ultra-fine tipped pencil that creates fine hair lines. Use upward strokes to match the direction of hair growth. Brow Wiz stays in place until washed off. Another good, cost-effective choice is *Define-A-Brow™* by Maybelline®, and slightly higher-priced *Brow Sculpting Marker™* by Laura Geller®.

*To reduce the look of puffy eyes, place wet *chamomile* or *green tea bags* in the refrigerator. In the morning apply the cooled tea bags onto eyes. The tannins in both teas reduce eye inflammation. Placing eye cream in the refrigerator works too. Apply the cool, refreshing cream under eyes in the morning.

*Another effective, anti-inflammatory eye treatment is *emu oil.* After just seven nightly applications, under eye puffiness will be resolved. I recommend continued nightly applications to maintain results. The bonus of emu oil is that it helps thicken thinning skin and smoothes lines and wrinkles too.

*To help reduce the look of dark circles, apply a drop of *castor oil* under each eye at bedtime. This oil absorbs, hydrates and plumps the delicate eye skin to help make the appearance of dark circles less noticeable. See my dark circle eliminator recipe made with potatoes in **More Beauty Recipes.**

*I'm a huge fan of **Eye Perfect** eye cream. It's affordable, yet powerful because it contains myriad properties that address eye issues. It contains resveratrol, skin firming antioxidants, hydrating squalane, and Matrixyl® and Argireline® peptides to help smooth and soften expression lines over time. Hyaluronic acid, collagen peptides, grape seed, minerals and amino acids prevent the breakdown of collagen. Super antioxidants alpha lipoic acid (ALA) and resveratrol nourish the delicate eye skin and protect against free radicals. The specialized formulation of DMAE firms and helps reduce puffiness within 20 minutes. Antioxidant alpha lipoic acid boosts the effects of DMAE. ALA gently exfoliates delicate skin around the eyes, reduces puffiness and brightens the eye area. Eye Perfect goes a long way. It's free of phthalates, petroleum and synthetic dyes, though contains trace parabens. As noted earlier, parabens in moderation are safe.

*I am also a fan of **Ultimate Eye Crème** with peptides, antioxidants and emu oil. This product contains no water. Emu oil is the first ingredient! As noted earlier, emu oil is transdermal so it pushes active ingredients deep down into the dermis past the epidermis, for faster results. Ultimate Eye Cream is free of parabens and phthalates.

*To improve eye muscle strength and fend off the need for reading glasses, consider wearing **pinhole glasses**. They are like regular glasses but are made of plastic and cost under $10 at most drug stores. The plastic lenses are riddled with dozens of small holes formed in a honeycomb pattern. When worn, the pattern of the holes block the peripheral rays of light from entering the pupils of the eyes. The minimized light forces the eyes to focus through <u>one</u> of the pinholes. Pinhole glasses supposedly strengthen the muscles of the eyes, though I have not found any studies that support this finding. However, I will tell you about an 80 year old body builder who introduced pinhole glasses to me. She revealed that since using pinhole glasses, she doesn't required reading glasses. So I bought a pair. That was over eight years ago, and to this day I don't require reading glasses either! I can thread a needle and read the fine print on the bottom of a lipstick tube with ease. Some individuals watch TV with them too. **NOTE:** Do not wear pinhole glasses outdoors, when driving or as a substitute for sunglasses.

*Dressing for success boosts our confidence. A great way to update your look is with a new pair of prescription glasses. Most Americans overpay for their glasses, even with vision benefit plans. If you wear glasses, you can purchase fashionable prescription eyewear online without compromising quality and pay a substantially lower price. **GlassesUSA®** eliminates the middleman and they don't outsource their work, which saves customers a lot of money. They process and ship each order in the shortest time span possible - all across the globe. They offer a large variety of frames, including designer brands. Their policy is to be in touch with the customer through every step of the way, making certain that prescriptions are correct - from preordering to after receiving your glasses. I have not been paid to endorse this brand. A cost-effective way to get your eyes tested is at Costco®.

See the above noted products and where to find them in **Safe, Effective Face & Body Product Suggestions.**

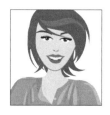

Age-Proofing Tip #40
Brighter Pearly Whites & Fresh Breath

A bright, white smile is one of the first things we notice about a person. And of course, fresh breath is a must! Below are several excellent suggestions that address healthy gums and teeth, cavity and plaque prevention, fresh breath and whiten teeth. These tips are sure to put a smile on your face!

*A basic routine should include brushing teeth both morning and evening, and flossing at least once a day. Use an extra soft toothbrush and brush very gently to prevent enamel abrasion and receding gums. Or use a **Sonicare®** tooth cleaning system.

*Be sure to invest in a new toothbrush every six months. Worn bristles can cause receding gums.

*Did you know that it takes only 12 hours for tartar to form on teeth? Flossing teeth at least once a day can prevent tartar buildup and bad breath. Many health experts agree that flossing supports heart health by removing harmful bacteria that can make their way into the bloodstream. Regular flossing will prevent inflammation of the gums (AKA gingivitis). Carry flossing sticks in a small zipper lock plastic sandwich bag when on the go. **NOTE:** Germs on hands and fingers can end up on dental floss causing a potential gum infection. Wash hands before flossing.

*I like waxed dental floss as it is less likely to fray between teeth. **Baking soda** on dental floss can help whiten between teeth where stains are the most difficult to reach. Make your own baking soda floss. **Here's what you do:**

Place two feet of waxed dental floss into 1 tsp. of baking soda. Coat it well, and then floss teeth. Wax helps the baking soda stick to the floss.

*For those with bleeding gums or prone to tarter or plaque buildup on teeth, **probiotics** can address the unfriendly bacteria in the mouth and help reduce red, inflamed, bleeding gums and plaque. **Here's what you do:**

Break open one or two probiotic capsules and apply the contents on a clean, extra soft toothbrush. Gently scrub the probiotics on teeth and gums. Close mouth and swish the probiotics around using your tongue to spread along the teeth and gums.

Do this for one to two minutes. Then either spit out or swallow the probiotics. Do not rinse your mouth. Oral probiotics help balance the flora in the digestive tract too!

*For brighter, whiter-looking teeth and to help remove tooth stains, try the tip below. **Here's what you do:**

Three times a week, sprinkle a little baking soda on a toothbrush, then apply toothpaste on top and brush teeth. Baking soda provides a gentle tooth, gum and mouth scrub for a bright smile, fresher breath and healthy gums.

*Yellow teeth are primarily caused by aging or consuming tooth-staining foods and drinks such as cola, tea, coffee, red wine and blueberries to name a few. It's impossible to brush after every drink or food we consume. Below is an effective, yet simple mouth rinse recipe that can quickly brighten your pearly whites when you're not able to brush. **Here's what you do:**

Combine 1 tbsp. water with 1 tbsp. oral grade hydrogen peroxide in a glass. Swish this mixture between teeth for about one to two minutes. Spit out the mixture and allow the peroxide bubbles to remain on teeth for another minute. Then rinse mouth with water. Your teeth will look instantly whiter.

*An article on *AOLHealth/HuffingtonPost* featured my strawberry whitening tip. Strawberries contain an enzyme called malic acid, which is found in many whitening toothpastes. The fiber in strawberries also helps remove bacteria from the teeth and mouth. **Here's what you do:**

Chew one strawberry and swish it around your mouth and between teeth for one to two minutes. Then swallow or spit out the mashed berry.

*Tooth bleaching kits such as **Crest 3D Whitestrips® with Advanced Seal** are a safe tooth whitening alternative. Crest 3D are my favorite whitening strips. They are enamel-safe and the strips stick very well onto teeth so there is no need to use messy gels or trays. For your first treatment, apply the white strips three days in a row for one hour. Leaving them on longer may cause a little tooth sensitivity. To maintain whiteness apply the strips bi-weekly or once a month. You may increase or reduce the number of treatments depending on how many tooth-staining foods you consume.

*To prevent stains and protect tooth enamel, drink tooth-staining or acidic beverages with a straw.

See the above noted products and where to find them in **Safe, Effective Face & Body Product Suggestions.**

Natural Breath Fresheners

Bad breath is often difficult to detect on ourselves so prevention is key. To keep bad breath in check, the following healthy tips can effectively remedy most causes.

*To prevent bad breath and reduce a cold, sore throat or flu, each morning scrape your tongue using a teaspoon. Actually, any type of stainless steel spoon will do the trick. **Here's what you do:**

Place the spoon (scoop down) onto the back of the tongue as far as you can go. Then scrape forward. Scraping removes bacteria from the back of the tongue where germs harbor.

*Sugar and artificial sweeteners such as sorbitol and malitol feed bacteria in the mouth, which causes cavities and bad breath. Natural sweetener **xylitol** helps banish bacteria and plaque by keeping the mouth moist. It can prevent cavities, tartar buildup and bad breath too. Though it sounds like a chemical ingredient, xylitol is a healthy sweetener that looks, tastes and measures like regular sugar. It is low-glycemic, all-natural, non-GMO, and lower in calories than regular sugar. It makes an excellent sugar substitute for those prone to tooth decay, yeast infections or diabetes. It can be incorporated with a low-carbohydrate diet. I like **XyloSweet®** brand. In addition, chewing xylitol gum is recommended for reducing plaque formation and freshening breath. Two brands that I like are **Cinnamon Spry®** and **Licorice XyliChew®.** They are gluten-free too.

*_Chlorella_ is loaded with chlorophyll which can effectively help eliminate bad breath. Chlorella is nutrient-packed freshwater green algae. It contains 19 essential amino acids that boost immunity as well as chlorophyll which offers powerful detoxifying properties to freshen breath, regulate bowel movements, support a healthy liver, and build red blood cells. Chlorella can eliminate heavy metals and offers many other anti-aging and health benefits. Add five to ten pellets to a protein smoothie or take the pellets with water after each meal of the day. Find out more about chlorella in **Age-Proofing Tip #51 - My Favorite Supplements for Women.**

*Drinking _green tea_ is another good way to help eliminate bad breath. Drink a cup after eating onions or garlic. It really does the trick! Green tea is also rejuvenating and can help with weight loss. See many more health tips about green tea in **Age-Proofing Tip #51 - My Favorite Supplements for Women.**

*Chewing on *fennel seeds* after eating a meal or snack can help eliminate bad breath. They can even help eliminate gas or bloating. Swallow or discard seeds after chewing.

*Post nasal drip, allergies, colds, sinus infections and dental surgery can cause bad breath. A *neti pot* gently washes away bacteria and mucus and is a safe, scientifically proven, drug-free method for relieving several causes of bad breath. Use a neti pot when feeling a cold, flu or sinus infection coming on, and during allergy season. **NOTE:** Be sure to use distilled water to ensure that no harmful bacteria is present. Be sure to clean the pot with soap and water before each use. Follow directions on the box to ensure proper use.

*_Peppermint tea_ can help drain the sinuses and calm inflamed nasal tissue. **Here's what you do:**

Boil 2 cups water in a sauce pan. Remove the pan from the stove and add 3-4 peppermint tea bags. Tie hair back, place a towel over your head and inhale the steaming peppermint vapor.

*Taking *oil of oregano* twice a day can help clear a sinus infection to improve breath. Follow the directions for usage on the bottle.

*_Grape-seed extract_ is an effective supplement that can help prevent post-nasal drip. Find it at a health food store and follow the directions for usage on the bottle.

*_Quercetin_ is a supplement that supports cardiovascular health, provides better breathing and helps prevent allergies. Find it at a health food store and follow the directions for usage on the bottle.

See the product noted above in **Safe, Effective Face & Body Product Suggestions.**

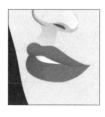

Age-Proofing Tip #41
Plumper Youthful-Looking Lips

Below I've noted several recipes, remedies and products for healthy, softer, more youthful-looking lips. The great news is we <u>can</u> naturally plump lips without the use of costly, painful injections.

Natural Lip Plumper – Peptides

As we age, our lips become thinner due to a reduction of collagen and hyaluronic acid (HA) production. Also, because lips do not have oil glands, they are vulnerable to dryness. When exposed to sun, wind, cold or heat, lips can become cracked, chapped, inflamed and sensitive.

Lips are primarily composed of connective tissue, collagen and HA. To safely plump and rejuvenate lips apply topical HA and peptides to naturally stimulate collagen and HA production. **Here's what you do:**

STEP 1: Gently exfoliate lips twice a week. This removes dry, chapped skin and allows lips to plump up when you apply peptides. Dip a soft toothbrush into some baking soda and scrub the lips in a gentle, circular motion. Then rinse and pat dry.

STEP 2: Each night, apply **Night Perfect Serum** or **Deep Penetrating LED Serum** on clean lips; then massage a drop of emu oil over either serum. Leave on overnight. Within two or three weeks lips will look more plump and smooth.

Night Perfect Serum (as noted above) is 100% peptides in a glycerin base. It is free of colors, parabens, flavor or fragrance (phthalates). **Deep Penetrating LED Serum** (peptides and HA in a water base) is also paraben and phthalate-free. You can also use this peptide with an LED Red Light Therapy unit. Apply the serum on lips and face prior to using an LED Red Light Therapy device. The deep penetrating lights help stimulate <u>collagen in the lips</u>, making them look plumper. They also soften lines and wrinkles around the lips including nasal labial folds and other wrinkles on the face. After the LED treatment, smooth a drop of **emu oil** on lips (and face) and leave on overnight. Emu oil is rich in omega 3s, 6s and 9s. As noted on earlier pages, emu oil is one-of-a-kind transdermal oil that pushes the active ingredients deep into the skin, or in this case, into the lips.

More Lip Tips

*In 2012 the media reported that over 400 lipstick brands contained <u>lead</u>! Also, whatever we place onto our lips, we ingest with every bite of food or drink we sip. Switch to all-natural, organic lip gloss and lipstick to ensure wellbeing. I like berry-tinted, red or pink lip gloss for moister, healthy lips. Unlined, glossy lips are more youthful and fresh-looking. You can find natural lip glosses at health food stores. Two of my favorite brands are **Aubrey Organics® Natural Lips** and **Bert's Bees®**. Both contain natural essential extracts and moisturizers.

A quick, natural lip tint recipe can be made with a pomegranate. **Here's what you do:**

Slice a fresh pomegranate in half. Using a cotton swab, absorb some of the pomegranate juice, and apply the red stain on clean lips. See more lip recipes in **More Beauty Recipes**.

*To help calm chapped, cracked, wind-burned lips, applying milk, honey and vitamin E are very soothing and healing. **Here's what you do:**

Dip a large cotton ball into 2-3 tbsp. warm milk and dab onto lips for three to five minutes. Milk contains lactic acid which exfoliates dry skin. The fat in milk moisturizes. Then, gently pat lips dry. Do not rinse lips. Next, apply a little raw honey on lips. Honey is a natural humectant that contains antibiotic properties to heal cracked, sensitive lips. Lastly, poke open a vitamin E capsule and apply its contents over the honey. Leave on overnight. Vitamin E hydrates and seals lips.

*__Black tea__ contains tannins that soften, moisturize and heal chapped or cracked lips. **Here's what you do:**

Apply a wet, warm, black tea bag on dry or cracked lips for 5 to 10 minutes. Then apply vitamin E or **Emu Oil Lip Balm**.

*The wax base of **Emu Oil Lip Balm** soothes and protects lips from wind and cold and provides a protective, thick coating which prevents chapped lips. This balm makes an excellent base for smoother lipstick application.

*Choose lip balms and lipsticks that contain hydrating ingredients such as cocoa and shea butter, honey, beeswax, glycerin, castor, primrose, olive or almond oil.

*__Mango__ contains enzymes that help exfoliate and plump. __Cayenne pepper__ stimulates circulation and also plumps. My lip plumping recipe is all-natural. However, do not try this if you have chapped or cracked lips. **Here's what you do:**

Combine 1 tbsp. mashed mango, ½ tsp. fresh lemon juice and a dash of cayenne pepper. Mash together and apply to lips for 2 minutes, then rinse. Afterward apply some un-petroleum jelly or moisturizing organic lip gloss.

*To make my healthy __un-petroleum jelly__ recipe, see **More Beauty Recipes.**

*Hormone changes and monthly menstruation can cause upper lip hair to darken and become more noticeable. I am not a fan of waxing because it removes natural peach fuzz and can cause ingrown hairs and clogged pores. When peach fuzz is waxed away, makeup slides off the skin causing a noticeably shiny upper lip. Instead of waxing, keep peach fuzz intact by clipping upper lip hair. During my modeling career, I did several close-up lip ads for photography, billboards, and TV commercials for lipsticks, balms and facial beauty products including Avon®, Dove®, and Revlon®, just to name a few. To date, I continue to clip my upper lip hair to keep it out of site. **NOTE:** Clipping lip hair does not cause thicker hair growth. That's an old wives tale. **Here's what you do:**

You will need a pair of cuticle scissors and a magnifying mirror. Stand in natural light by a window and use the fine, curved tip portion of the scissors to very carefully clip long, dark lip hair. Don't rush it. Take your time to ensure that you don't clip skin. Do this once a week.

Mouth Line Eliminators

*Exfoliating the area around the mouth regularly can help reduce mouth lines. An enzyme mask can help. Below is my *Mouth Line Eliminator Mask* recipe. It's a highly effective way to help soften and smooth mouth lines. **Here's what you do**:

Rub the inside peel of a ripe papaya around mouth and on lips. Apply it on clean face too. The moist enzymes will dry in about 15-20 minutes. Then rinse with tepid water. Papaya is a natural alternative to Retin-A. Top skin care salons charge $65 to $85 for papaya enzyme masks. Do this yourself for under $3.

*After making the recipe noted above, apply peptides or EGF with peptides and antioxidants on the skin. These powerful skin care products help nourish and repair, hydrate and plump fine lines and wrinkles around the mouth and on the face. Some of my favorite products are **Ultimate Age-Proofing Complex** (with peptides, EGF and antioxidants) or **Uplift Serum** (peptides & antioxidants), **De-Aging Solution** (with EGF, antioxidants and squalane), **Beyond Essential** (Peptides & Antioxidants). Night-time choices are **Night Perfect Serum** or **Deep Penetrating LED Serum** with **emu oil** on top to push active ingredients deep into the dermis.

*Topical hyaluronic acid (HA) serum or mist binds moisture to skin to increase hydration in the skin. HA is a natural moisture *magnet* for dry, thirsty skin, binding up to 1000 times its weight in water. It's a powerful topical supplement that can plump wrinkles around the mouth. Effective products that contain HA are **Hyaluronic Hydrating Mist, De-Aging Solution**, **Ultimate Age-Proofing Complex, Refill Wrinkle Filler** and **Uplift Serum**. When taken as an oral supplement, HA can effectively plump wrinkles, thin lips, lines around the mouth, and hydrate the eyes, joints, scalp and more. HA is noted in many sections throughout these pages.

See the above noted products and where to find them in **Safe, Effective Face & Body Product Suggestions.**

Canker Sore Relief

Stress is the main cause of canker sores. The following suggestions and remedies can provide relief.

*To reduce stress try **Rescue Remedy® by Bach**, an oral homeopathic aid that provides speedy relief during stressful times. I like the Original Flowers Essences as a tincture or spray. Apply 4 drops under the tongue. **NOTE:** Do not take this remedy if breastfeeding or pregnant. It contains some alcohol. Find Rescue Remedy® at health food stores. See more tips on how to address and reduce stress in **Age-Proofing Tip #6 - Managing Stress for Better Health, Rejuvenation & Weight Loss** and perform my two-minute ritual noted in **Age-Proofing Tip #7 - 'Waist' Management De-stressing Ritual.**

*Avoid consuming acidic or spicy foods until the canker sore heals.

***Propolis** is therapeutic glue-like substance created by bees. It is derived from tree and plant sap and is rich in anti-inflammatory and antibiotic properties. When applied topically or taken orally, it is known to help remedy canker sores.

*Taking acidophilus on an empty stomach can help remedy canker sores. If you don't have any acidophilus on hand, yogurt will work. Placing plain yogurt onto canker sores can soothe inflammation and pain. **Here's what you do:**

Swish plain yogurt in your mouth in the area of the canker sore for a minute or two. Then swallow or spit out. Do not rinse mouth.

*Another proven remedy that can help calm a canker sore is black tea. **Here's what you do:**

Dab the canker sore with a moistened black tea bag. Tannins in tea can help reduce inflammation.

***Chamomile** is a known antibacterial that helps reduce painful, inflamed cold sores. **Here's what you do:**

Boil ¼ cup of water and add 2 chamomile tea bags. Let steep and cool to room temperature. Do not drink the tea, but rather swish it throughout the mouth on the canker sore area.

See the above noted products and where to find them in **Safe, Effective Face & Body Product Suggestions.**

Cold Sore Prevention & Relief

One of the best ways to prevent an outbreak of herpes I and II is to avoid stress. Stress can weaken the immune system. During an outbreak, be sure to consult with your physician. In the meantime, the following remedies have been known to help provide relief and help strengthen immune health. **NOTE:** Check with your health care professional for medical advice or before taking supplements.

*Stress can cause a herpes outbreak. If you feel tense or anxious, **_Rescue Remedy_**® can provide quick relief of stress or anxiety attacks. Read more about it in the previous section, **Canker Sores.** Find it at health food stores.

*Getting sufficient sleep is essential to keeping the immune system strong.

***_Dry-brushing_** the body can help improve blood circulation and immunity. Brush up toward the heart to increase blood flow. Much of the natural flow of blood is at the base of the spine and pelvis so dry brushing that area is particularly helpful.

*Regular exercise oxygenates the blood. Oxygen kills pathogens.

*Maintain a balanced pH. Diet influences pH. The more acidic the pH, the higher chance of having an outbreak, so it is best to switch to an alkaline diet. Alkaline foods include fresh, raw green leafy vegetables and salads, legumes, potatoes, fresh vegetable juices, whole grains and low-glycemic fruits. Add antioxidant-rich powdered greens to a protein shake or take chlorella pellets after meals. As noted on previous pages, chlorella is an immune-boosting green algae. Chlorella provides many benefits which is why it's been noted several times throughout these pages.

*Avoid sugar, refined and processed foods such as white flour products, rice, crackers, cakes, cookies, corn syrup, dairy products, all meats including hot dogs, sausage, cold cuts, burgers, fish, shellfish, chicken, vinegar, ketchup, mayonnaise, pickles, spicy foods, hot sauce, saturated fats, hydrogenated oils, margarine, alcohol, soft drinks, juices, black tea and coffee. There are many books available in health food stores that address balancing your pH with diet.

***Garlic** or odorless **Kyolic®** brand capsules contain over 200 disease-fighting compounds which can help prevent certain viruses, infections, colds, flu, herpes I and herpes II and can fight bacteria, parasites, yeast overgrowth and fungus. Garlic has no known side effects and is safe to use on a long-term basis. NOTE: If taking blood thinning meds, check with your doctor before taking garlic supplements. Read more health benefits of garlic in **Age-Proofing Tip #53 - Super Foods**.

***Vitamin D3** is an excellent supplement that helps calm stress and helps reduce outbreaks. Read many more benefits of Vitamin D3 in **Age-Proofing Tip #51 - My Favorite Supplements for Women.**

*Taking a **vitamin C** supplement can help calm inflammation and address the herpes virus. Choose a non-acidic vitamin C such as ester or buffered C which is fat-soluble.

***Olive leaf extract** and **grape seed extract** can help keep herpes in check. Olive leaf extract contains anti-viral, antifungal and antibacterial agents. Grape seed extract is a powerful antioxidant.

*Systemic enzymes are known to help destroy the protein coat of the herpes virus. An excellent and affordable brand of systemic enzymes is **Dr. Wong's Essentials Zymessence®.** NOTE: Though less costly and very powerful, Zymessence® is not suitable for vegans or vegetarians. **Vitalzyme X** is another brand of systematic enzymes for vegans and vegetarians.

Omega 3-fatty acids such as *flaxseed oil* and **turmeric** (curcumin) can help fight inflammation. Take these supplements twice to three times a day with meals. Read more benefits of these supplements in **Age-Proofing Tip #51 - My Favorite Supplements for Women.**

Topical Products Suggestions for Herpes

Olive Gold 03 suspends super oxygen molecules in ozonated olive oil, allowing deep penetration into skin. It contains natural anti-bacterial, antifungal and antiviral properties that can be applied to herpes sores and used for myriad applications including cuts, burns, rashes and eczema.

*As noted in the canker sore section, propolis is a powerful topical and oral aid that can remedy many types of sores. *Propolis* is a therapeutic glue-like substance that is created by bees. It is derived from the gummy substance produced by trees and plants and is rich in anti-inflammatory and antibiotic properties. When applied topically or taken orally, it is known to help reduce herpes sores.

*An English study reveals that *pure lavender essential oil* can help speed heal cold sores. Another expert on herpes suggests that combining lavender with tea tree oil makes an excellent soothing, herpes healer for genital herpes. **Here's what you do:**

Combine 3 drops pure lavender essential oil with 1 drop pure tea tree oil and ½ tsp. squalane oil. Apply mixture on the sores.

Echinacea is a well known immune booster. Applying *echinacea* directly on the sores and take it as an oral tincture 4-5 times a day during a herpes outbreak.

See where to find the products noted above in **Safe, Effective Face & Body Product Suggestions.**

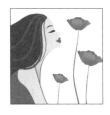

Age-Proofing Tip #42
Hormone Balance

When it comes to menopause, no two women are alike. Our lifestyles affect our output of testosterone, estrogen, and progesterone levels which can vary from day to day. Those who live a quiet, less hectic lifestyle may breeze through menopause. Other women, with more hectic schedules, may experience a different outcome due to sleeplessness, stress or adrenal exhaustion.

As our body chemistry changes, shifts in hormones and dietary needs occur. Taking natural herbs such as dong quai, chaste tree, and valerian root tea may have helped your sister or best friend, but these alternatives may not necessarily work for you. The good news is that many studies reveal that the foods we consume, the skin and body care products we apply, and physical activities we incorporate can be very helpful during this special time.

TIP: Menopause is perfectly natural, so choosing to embrace this passage rather than dreading it may be the best approach. Attitude is everything and education is power. Read all you can about the stages of menopause so you know what to expect and your loved ones will better understand too. Two great books are *"The Complete Idiots Guide to Hormone Weight Loss"* by Dr. Alicia Stanton and *"The Hormone Diet"* by Natasha Turner, a leading Canadian Naturopath. Learn more online at InternationalHormoneSociety.com.

Helpful Advice from Real Women

I love to talk with women who have gone through this passage of life. I was fortunate to speak with women between the ages of 52 and 62. Almost every one of them experienced few uncomfortable signs. I was happy to learn that they had all incorporated several of the tips that I've noted throughout these pages. Below, I've provided some additional helpful tips that the gals shared with me. However, it is always best to have a conversation with your health care professional before implementing dietary and supplement changes.

*Apply body products that are free of phthalates and parabens to avoid hormonal disruption, rashes, allergies and more. Phthalates are synthetic fragrances that are known carcinogens and can affect our mood, hormones and physical health. They are found in scented face and body lotions, creams, shampoos, hairsprays, deodorants, toothpaste, candles, laundry detergents and household cleansers. Parabens are preservatives. Read more in **Age-Proofing Tip #11 - Avoid Parabens**, **Tip #12 - Avoid Phthalates** and **Tip #13 - Switch to Healthy Household Cleaners.**

*A low-carbohydrate diet is best during this stage of life. This way of eating naturally balances hormones, promotes a feeling of wellbeing, prevents inflammation, helps slow aging, and prevents weight gain.

*Consume colorful pesticide-free vegetables and low-glycemic fruits, soy products, nuts and whey protein. Reduce red meat or switch to grass-fed beef. It is higher in good omega fatty acids and lower in fat.

*Consume high fiber foods to help remove toxins, balance hormones and prevent constipation. Drink 10-12 glasses of water per day when eating high fiber foods. This prevents gas and bloating.

*Soy, lentil, lima and kidney beans contain phytoestrogens called isoflavones, which act like the body's natural estrogen to stabilize and help suppress hot flashes. Eat one to two servings of phytoestrogen-rich foods daily including soy beans, roasted soy nuts, soy cheese, soy yogurt, soy milk (have a soy latte), and tofu.

*Some women experience excess estrogen in their system. In this case **calcium D-glucarate** supplements can help balance the production of estrogen. It's particularly beneficial to women with hormone imbalances or a history of breast cancer. Foods rich in calcium D-glucarate are apples, broccoli, citrus fruits, and cherries.

*Add **whey protein** to morning smoothies. Whey is high in protein, antioxidants, and glutathione to help build lean muscle mass and support the immune system. See my low-glycemic blueberry smoothie made with whey powder in **My Favorite Healthy Meal and Snack Recipes. NOTE:** Whey powder can cause bloating and gas for many individuals. Hemp protein powder is a non-bloating protein alternative.

*Take flaxseed oil or evening primrose oil to help balance hormones, slow aging, ignite fat burning, and help keep skin youthful and supple. They are rich in omega 3s. Other good omega 3s are fresh fish, sardines, avocados, and walnuts.

*Vitamin B supplements can help reduce stress, support healthy skin, hair, muscle tone and uplift mood. **Vitamin B5** (pantothenic acid) supports the adrenal system. Approximately 300 to 500 mg a day is suggested.

*A recent study revealed that over 80% of women in the USA are deficient in **vitamin D.** Vitamin D regulates the release of insulin, supports our weight loss goals, uplifts the mood, prevents depression, and is known to lower breast and other cancer risks by 50%, and much more. Generally, a minimum of 1,000 mg of vitamin D daily is recommended for menopausal women. However, many women require even more. Have your doctor check for vitamin D levels. Read more about vitamin D in **Age-Proofing Tip #51 - My Favorite Supplements for Women.**

*To naturally balance hormones, increase energy, uplift mood, strengthen nails, and improve the look of skin and hair, take **chlorella** three times a day. It's a *super* green algae that can clear hormonal adult acne and heavy metals from the system. Take 5-10 chlorella pellets after meals or crush and add to a whey or hemp protein smoothie. Read more about chlorella in **Age-Proofing Tip #51 - My Favorite Supplements for Women.**

*Take 1,000-2,000 milligrams of buffered **vitamin C** to support the immune system, calm inflammation, prevent and speed recovery from disease, prevent bruising and improve skin texture. Eat at least five to eight servings of vitamin C-rich fruits and vegetables. Find many choices in **Age-Proofing Tip #53 - Super Foods**.

*To avoid hot flashes, stop smoking and avoid caffeine, spicy food, and alcohol in the afternoon or evening. Alcohol interferes with our natural production of HGH when at rest.

*Get eight hours of uninterrupted sleep to help increase production of HGH. Avoid watching the evening news or violent TV shows prior to bed time. They cause anxiety, negative thoughts, and sleeplessness. Perform a calming pre-bed ritual. Drink a cup of soothing hibiscus or valerian tea and take time to pray or meditate. A calming bath is helpful too. See my recipes in **Age-Proofing Tip #46 - Bath & Body.**

*Vitamin B6 is best taken at night for calming and helps reduce cortisol production. Both **5-HTP** and melatonin are drug-free natural choices that can help induce sleep. Taking a **melatonin** supplement shuts off cortisol when sleeping. This can help with weight loss. Read more about 5-HTP and melatonin in **Age-Proofing Tip #16 - Importance of Rejuvenating Sleep.**

*Osteoporosis is a major concern for women, especially as we age. **Calcium citrate** offers a unique delivery system that is readily absorbed by the body while at rest. Calcium prevents bone disease, joint problems, and loss of collagen. Combine calcium supplements with magnesium at bedtime to relax muscles, induce sleep, prevent muscle twitching (restless legs), prevent grinding of teeth, and regulate the bowels. **Magnesium** improves endurance and strength. Calcium is often combined with magnesium. One brand I like is by Solary®. Read about **Body Vibration Plates** for preventing bone loss in **Age-Proofing Tip #58.**

*Overweight, post-menopausal women with breast cancer experience higher hormone levels that trigger more aggressive breast cancer tumor growth if they sleep less than seven hours nightly. It is imperative for all women to get eight uninterrupted hours of sleep.

*Jogging or running marathons are not considered good for the adrenal glands or joints. Incorporate daily calming exercise such as peaceful walking, yoga, Pilates, and stretching. Lifting weights two to three times weekly helps build muscle tone and speeds fat burning.

*By the time we reach our 30s our bodies produce less natural HGH. Amino acids play an essential role in building protein and maintaining hormone health, especially for those who are feeling or appear older than their years. **Meditropin®** is an amino acid-rich effervescent drink mix that can energize, nourish, repair and rejuvenate the body. The amino acids help the body to *naturally* stimulate HGH production. Meditropin® is not a steroid or HGH so it is a safe alternative to costly HGH injections which are known to have side-effects. Meditropin® can help nourish the adrenal and pituitary glands for hormonal support. When combined with a low carbohydrate diet, Meditropin® uplifts mood and energy, provides a restful sleep, improves muscle tone, increases libido and much more. It is used worldwide. Women going through menopause can greatly benefit from Meditropin®. Take it five nights a week for three consecutive months. Check with your health care professional before ordering this product. **NOTE:** Not recommended for vegetarians or vegans as it contains porcine and fish.

*Take some **you** time during lunch and dinner breaks. Eat meals with all electronic gadgets turned off, including your cell phone, to reduce stress and halt cortisol production.

*Deep breathing is important. Perform my de-stressing ritual every hour while at work. See how to do it in **Age-Proofing Tip #7 - 'Waist' Management De-stressing Ritual.**

*When feeling stressed during the day, try ***Rescue Remedy***®, a homeopathic calming tonic. It's a blend of herbal flowers and plants. Read more about it **Age-Proofing Tip #9 - Brain Boosters & Good Mood Foods.**

*Chinese acupuncture is a natural, drug-free treatment that can help balance hormones and other challenges associated with menopause such as loss of libido, backache, fatigue, graying hair, hair loss and vaginal dryness.

*To address vaginal dryness and as a healthy, effective personal lubricant use ***squalane oil*** derived from olives. It is 100% natural and free of phthalates, parabens, and petroleum. Unlike many personal lubricants on the market, squalane oil is not sticky and does not sting. It is perfect for sensitive or irritated skin.

*Unlike conventional saunas, ***FIR infrared sauna blankets*** can speed weight loss and eliminate toxins by heating subcutaneous fat. In addition, they stimulate circulation, eliminate heavy metals, curb appetite, reduce stress, and increase fat burning. In fact, for several hours after having had a FIR infrared treatment, the core of the body continues to burn fat! Hormone health doctor, Alicia Stanton, and countless others recommend FIR infrared treatments for hormone balance. I've been promoting this treatment for some time. One session can cost between $18 and $40 at a spa. Find out more about the weight loss and health benefits and how you can purchase a FIR infrared sauna blanket valued at $900 for under $300 in **Age-Proofing Tip #59 - FIR Infrared Sauna Blankets. Note:** Prices are subject to change.

*For those who are not able to attend exercises classes, or are challenged with fibromyalgia or asthma, daily use of a body vibration plate can help balance hormones, improve mood, rapidly tone muscles, prevent bone loss, reduce 'muffin tops', cellulite, speed weight loss and much more. Find out more about this phenomenal home unit in **Age-Proofing Tip #58 - Body Vibration Plates.**

*Focus on staying positive and living life to the fullest. Make life an adventure.

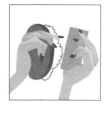

Age-Proofing Tip #43
Hand Rejuvenating Tips

Our hands are vulnerable to everyday environmental exposure. From the sun's UV rays and using household cleaning products, to changing diapers and playing sports, our hands can age very quickly - if we don't pay attention to them. In addition, the hands produce less natural oils than the rest of the body, so hydration is important. The following age-proofing tips will help keep your hands looking beautiful and more youthful.

*Drink 8-10 glasses of water a day and take omega 3 fatty acids such as flaxseed oil. Read about additional benefits of omega 3s in **Age-Proofing Tip #51 - My Favorite Supplements for Women.**

*Did you know that frequently immersing hands in water damages and weaken nails, causes splitting and peeling, strips hands of moisture, and may be one of the main causes of arthritis in joints of the hands? Be sure to wear lined rubber gloves when doing laundry, handling cleaning products, washing fruits and veggies or doing dishes.

*For those challenged with splitting or peeling nails, massage them with olive or emu oil and leave on overnight.

*Alpha hydroxy acid (AHA) cream can help remove yellow stains from nails and age spots from tops of hands. The beauty of AHA cream is that is gently exfoliates while it deeply moisturizes so it won't dry out nails or hands. Follow this nightly regimen for three weeks, then twice weekly for maintenance, and you'll be left with healthy-looking nails and spot-free, younger-looking hands. **Here's what you do:**

Massage some AHA cream such as **Evenly Radiant Overnight Peel** on each nail prior to bedtime. Also massage the tops of hands with the AHA cream to help reduce the look of age spots.

*Another excellent method of reducing yellow, stained or rippled nails is by buffing them with a gentle ***Revlon® Crazy Shine Nail Buffer***. It makes nails look 400% shinier without the use of nail polish. It's simple and fast. **Here's what you do:**

Buff each nail with the light green side of the buffer. Then use the flip side of the buffer to polish nails to an incredible shine.

*Milk is an excellent hand rejuvenator. **Here's what you do:**

Once a week, place hands in a bowl of warm milk and soak for 15 minutes. The lactic acid in milk exfoliates skin and fades age spots, while the fat moisturizes. Milk also softens cuticles and chapped, dry hands.

*Do you have dry cuticles? **Here's what you do:**

After soaking hands in milk as noted above, massage olive oil into nails and cuticles. Gently push cuticles back using a wooden cuticle stick. **NOTE:** Do not cut cuticles as they protect nail beds from infection.

*If you are experiencing thinning skin on hands, this tip will help thicken the skin and rejuvenate the look of hands. **Here's what you do:**

At bedtime, apply your choice of antioxidant or peptide-rich cream or serum on hands. Then apply and massage 2-3 drops emu oil on top. Leave on overnight. Emu oil pushes the active ingredients of the antioxidants and/or peptides deep down to the dermis of the skin for faster results.

The following knuckle and cuticle 'eraser' instantly rejuvenates the look of hands. **Here's what you do:**

Massage ***Neutrogena® Natural Lip Balm*** or ***Emu Lip Balm*** on knuckles and cuticles. The natural wax and oils in these lip products instantly smooth the look of wrinkled-looking knuckles and banish dry cuticles.

*Another knuckle-smoothing option is buffing them lightly using the finest grit of a 4-way buffing/filing block. Moisturize afterward with natural ***Anti-Aging Hand Crème*** or ***Skinlasting Super Hydrator.***

*Carrying heavy items like grocery bags or lifting heavy weights creates blood flow to the veins in the hands. This causes the veins to protrude which is often associated with aged-looking hands. Whenever possible, use a shopping cart to transport groceries, boxes or heavy bags. To address protruding veins, an experienced phlebologist (vein specialist) can perform sclerotherapy. This involves a series of injections that contain a saline formulation that collapses and dissolves the veins.

*I recommend and personally use ***LED Red Light Therapy*** on my hands to prevent age spots and wrinkled knuckles. It's one of my secret weapons for my youthful-looking hands. I still get calls to double my hands for actresses and models who are much younger than I am.

Nail Disorders

Lack of certain vitamins or nutrients, dark nail polish colors, allergies, drug reactions, smoking, lupus, thyroid problems, lung, liver or kidney disease, cancer, psoriasis, eczema, or warts can affect nail color and texture. I've noted some safe options below. However, I recommend seeing a physician to discuss treatment for persistent nail challenges.

*Nail breakage and peeling or brittle nails may be an indication that you are low in trace minerals copper and manganese as well as essential fatty acids, calcium, zinc, protein, biotin, vitamin A, B6 and B12. See the list of **Nail Enriching Foods** below. I strongly recommend wearing rubber gloves when using household cleaners to protect nails. In addition, condition nails nightly with either olive oil, coconut or emu oil. Another option is vitamin E. Apply some un-petroleum jelly on top of the oil(s), put on some gloves and wear them overnight to keep in moisture. See my recipe for un-petroleum jelly in **More Beauty Recipes.**

*For weak nails or those that grow slowly, consider taking silica gel which can help strengthen nails and speed growth. Prenatal vitamins can also speed nail growth. Biotin supplements and biotin-rich foods increase the thickness of nails. See **Nail Enriching Foods** below.

*Nail fungus can take several months to remedy. Gray or brown colored nails may be a sign of fungus. Oral anti-fungal medications should be used as a last resort as they can be extremely hard on the liver, and require doctor's supervision. Applying a topical anti-fungal product such as tea tree oil or **Vick's® Vapor Rub** on toe nails is known to help reduce mild cases of nail fungus. **NOTE:** If fungus persists, seek the advice of a physician. A temporary topical is grapefruit seed extract. **Here's what you do:**

Dilute 2 drops grapefruit seed extract (GSE) with 1 tsp. coconut oil and massage into nails. I recommend **NutriBiotic® Grapefruit Seed Extract**.

*Pitted or bumpy nails may be caused by eczema, warts or psoriasis. Try lightly buffing nails with a **Revlon® Crazy Shine Nail Buffer.** It smoothes lines and shines nails. You may also use the smoothest grit of a four-sided nail buffer. At bedtime, massage nails with castor, olive or emu oil and follow with vitamin E. Massage into hands too. Put on some cotton gloves and leave on overnight.

*Ridges are a sign of normal aging or can be an indication of poor absorption of vitamins and minerals. Use a ridge filling base coat to create smooth looking nails or a **Revlon® Crazy Shine Nail Buffer**.

*Pale nails may indicate anemia. You may need more iron. See the **Nail Enriching Foods** noted in this section.

*Grey or beige nails may be a result of taking antibiotics or that you may need more vitamin B12. See **Nail Enriching Foods**.

*Yellow nails may be a result of wearing dark polish, smoking or applying self-tanning creams and hair products that stain. Lung disease may also cause yellow nails. See your personal physician to be certain.

*Pink or white areas on nails are due to trauma or you may need more zinc in your diet. Did you bump your finger? This could also be a sign of an underlying kidney problem. See your personal physician to be certain.

Nail Enriching Foods

Proper nutrition can strengthen and smooth nails. Healthy oils, nuts and seeds found in omega 3s, plant-based 6s, and 9s contain essential fatty acids that improve nails, hair, skin and overall wellbeing. A diet rich in calcium, biotin, protein, iron, beta carotene, vitamins A, B, C, E, and zinc can address many nail issues. These nutrients are found in a variety of yellow, orange, green and red fruits, vegetables, grains, and leafy greens. Below are beneficial foods for healthy nails.

-Calcium-rich foods include low-fat cheese and milk, butter, tofu, sesame seeds, sardines, dark leafy vegetables, carrots and fresh carrot juice. Take calcium supplements daily.

-Biotin-rich foods include cereals, milk, egg yolks, peanut butter, lentils and cauliflower. Biotin supplements are recommended.

-Iron-rich foods include spinach, kale, dark leafy greens, liver and raisins.

-Protein-rich foods include tofu, eggs, chicken, turkey, quail, lamb, salmon, sardines, mackerel, tuna, duck, goose, venison, lean grass-fed beef, liver, whey or soy protein powder, nut butters, and beans.

-Beta carotene-rich foods include yellow and orange peppers, carrots, red and orange tomatoes, watermelon, sweet potatoes, papaya, broccoli, spinach and leafy green vegetables.

-Healthy seeds and nuts are rich in oils that hydrate and improve the condition of skin, hair and nails. Nuts include almonds, walnuts, pecans, pistachios and macadamias. Healthy seeds are flax, pumpkin and sunflower. Healthy oils rich in omega 3s are found in avocados, flaxseed oil and fresh fish. Healthy plant-based omega 6s and 9s are found in grape seed, olive, pumpkin, safflower, sunflower, and evening primrose oils. These oils also help ignite fat-burning and balance hormones.

-Vitamin A-rich foods include sweet potatoes, carrots, spinach, kale, egg yolks, oysters and non-fat milk.

-Vitamin B-rich foods include *dark* leafy greens, red meat, turkey, chicken, butter, eggs, peanut butter, bananas, whole grains, fish, milk, cheese, yogurt and vitamin B supplements.

-Vitamin C-rich foods include cantaloupe, strawberries, tomatoes, red peppers, citrus fruits and green peas.

-Vitamin E-rich foods include wild salmon, lean meats, almonds, almond butter, peanut butter, sunflower seeds, leafy greens, olives, olive and sesame oil, legumes and vitamin E supplements.

-Zinc-rich foods include eggs, liver and milk. Take 25 mg zinc supplements daily. Check with your doctor before taking supplements.

Natural 5-Step Manicure

As a top hand and parts model for celebrities, keeping my nails long and healthy is important. You'll love my natural manicure for beautiful, strong, naturally shiny nails.

Ingredients:
1 tsp. almond or olive oil
1 cup milk (skim, 1% or 2%)
1 orange wood stick
1 buffing block
1 four-way nail file
1 tsp. distilled white vinegar
1 cotton ball
1 Revlon® Crazy Shine Nail Buffer

1. Apply half the olive or almond oil on nails and massage them for 30 seconds. Place milk in a glass bowl and warm in the microwave for 30 seconds. Make certain the milk is warm - not hot. Soak hands in milk for 10 minutes. Rinse with tepid water and pat dry.

2. Massage hands and nails with the remaining oil for 2 minutes. Wrap an orangewood stick with cotton and gently push cuticles back.

3. Trim nails by gently filing them in a back and forth motion using the medium grit side of a four-way nail file. Shape nails using the medium grit as well.

4. Saturate a cotton ball with white vinegar and wipe over each fingernail. Vinegar balances the pH of the nails. Allow the vinegar to dry for five minutes.

Nail Polish Application Tips

Using nail polish remover can strip and weaken nails. If you like to paint your nails regularly, the following tips can help make nail polish last longer.

Ingredients:
1 bottle of nail polish remover
2-3 cotton balls
1 tbsp. distilled white vinegar
1 bottle nail polish
1 can of cooking spray

1. After removing polish with nail polish remover, wash hands with soap and water.

2. Apply distilled white vinegar on nails with a cotton ball. Let the vinegar dry (about five minutes) before applying fresh nail polish. White vinegar balances the pH of nails. It also helps nail polish stay on longer.

3. Next, apply 2 thin coats of nail polish. Allow at least 3 minutes for each coat to dry.

4. To speed-dry polish, apply cooking spray on nails. Choose from natural olive oil or non-GMO canola oil. The oil also helps banish dry-looking cuticles.

NOTE: Many nail polishes contain phthalates which are known to affect our health and hormones. Find organic phthalate-free nail polish brands noted in **Safe, Effective Face & Body Product Suggestions.**

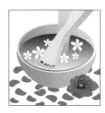

Age-Proofing Tip #44
Fabulous Feet

One of the main causes of cracked heels is walking barefoot and wearing sandals or back-less shoes. In particular, walking barefoot on flat surfaces places extreme pressure on the fat pads of the heels causing them to flatten out, spread and crack.

Another common cause of cracked heels is using a callous blade. Within days of removing skin with a blade, the heel skin grows back quickly and becomes even thicker than before, re-sulting in more cracks. The reason for faster, thicker skin growth is because the body's natural repair mode triggers when excessive skin is removed. The body responds by rushing even more new cells to the area. See a safer way to reduce thick heal skin below.

If experiencing deep, bleeding heel cracks or pain when walking, this may be a sign of diabetes. Diabetics are prone to very dry, cracked heels because they have more difficulty producing oil. Athletes' foot may be another reason for cracked heels. See your physician if cracked heels or pain persists. The following tips can help remedy many foot issues including cracked heels.

*Never walk barefoot in the house. Wear thick socks or slippers to cushion the fat pads of the heels. This prevents cracked heels. In the winter I recommend wearing socks *and* slippers at home.

*Hydrate your body. Drink eight glasses of water a day, and in-clude a diet rich in omega 3 fatty acids such as flaxseeds and oil, walnuts, <u>fresh</u> fish and plant-based omega 6 oils such as avocados, evening primrose and almonds. Omega 9-rich olive oil is also recommended.

*Each morning after showering, apply a penetrating moisturizer on feet. I recommend and personally use natural **Zim's® Crack Crème.** It's made with natural hydrating ingredients including glycerin, myrcia oil and arnica extract. Zim's® hydrates dry cu-ticles and banishes cracked heels instantly so feet are soft and look pretty year round.

*For extremely thick, deeply cracked heels try this helpful tip. Using a foot file, lightly file dry heels. Rinse feet off and pat them dry. Afterward, apply some cortizone ointment on heels, put on some socks and leave on overnight. Do this for three nights in a row and heels with be noticeably smoother. To maintain soft, crack-free heals, follow the three previous tips and incorporate the suggested products.

*Below is an excellent foot bath recipe that exfoliates and hydrates cracked, dry heels. **Here's what you do:**

Combine ½ gallon cold milk and ½ gallon hot water in a foot bath or large plastic basin and soak feet for 15 minutes. The lactic acid in milk softens and gently exfoliates cracked heels. Rinse and pat feet dry. Apply some shea or cocoa butter on feet, wrap them with cellophane, and put on some socks. After 45 minutes, remove the cellophane, and massage the butter into feet. Re-apply the socks and wear them overnight.

Visit www.youtube.com/user/BeautyGuru/videos online and see **More Beauty Recipes** on latter pages. Check with your physician before trying new ingredients or products.

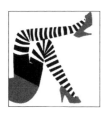

Age-Proofing Tip #45
Gorgeous Gams

When it comes to legs, one of the main concerns of many women is cellulite. I have wonderful news! You've probably read that cellulite is hereditary. If your mother has it, you'll have it too. Not true! Don't let the myths discourage you. With some simple, but consistent techniques, you can dramatically smooth and reduce the look of cellulite.

Everyone has cellulite - even babies! As we age, collagen fibers under the skin and around fat cells become trapped with lymphatic fluids and toxins. As years go by, poor circulation and breakdown of collagen causes more fluids and toxins to build, forcing their way up through the connective tissues. This weakens the tissue and congests the lymphatic system causing unsightly 'dimples.' Cellulite becomes more noticeable in our 30s and 40s because estrogen and collagen production begins to fluctuate. This causes the surface layers of the skin to thin and lose elasticity.

It probably took 20 plus years for your cellulite to develop, so consistency and patience is the key to achieving visibly dramatic results. The following tips can improve the look of cellulite.

*Exfoliating the thighs stimulates collagen production and regenerates new, fresh cells to the surface. This also triggers the production of elastin, making the skin firmer and thicker. In addition, exfoliating cellulite-prone areas releases toxins and fluids, ensuring smoother looking thighs.

*Dry brushing gently removes surface layers of dead skin and increases the blood flow within the subcutaneous fat layer, detoxifying and smoothing the skin. The motion of dry brushing boosts circulation which helps drain the lymphatic system and releases the body of toxins and excess fluids. This promotes internal cleansing. In Japan, dry brushing is routine hygiene for all women. Dry brushes are made with natural bristles or palm plants. The Japanese palm brush is slightly more abrasive and can be used on dry or wet skin. **NOTE:** Avoid dry brushing tender skin or areas that have cuts or rashes. **Here's what you do:**

Dry brushing is best done a.m. and p.m. prior to showering. Stand in front of a mirror and inspect the arms, thighs, buttocks and tummy for signs of cellulite. Dry brush each area for 30 seconds to 1 minute. If you have more time, take an extra few minutes to include an overall body brushing. The best technique for dry brushing is brushing up toward the heart in a semi-circle motion. Start at the hands and brush up to the shoulders. Next, start at the ankles and brush up to the top of the upper thighs. Then brush the buttocks and stomach up toward the heart. Skin should be slightly pink - not red. After dry brushing take a dry sauna or lay in a FIR infrared sauna blanket. Then shower. Read more about **FIR infrared sauna blankets** as an effective toxin reducer, weight loss and pain management therapy in **Age-Proofing Tip #59**.

*Another exfoliating option is a body scrub. While in the shower, sprinkle baking soda on a wet face cloth, or make my body salt scrub recipe below. Concentrate on scrubbing thighs and other cellulite-prone areas. **Here's what you do:**

Combine 1 cup Morton® or sea salt with ¼ cup almond or olive oil. Store the mixture in a BPA-free plastic container and keep it in the shower. After cleansing skin, turn shower off and apply the scrub onto cellulite-prone areas. Scrub each area for 30 seconds in a gentle, circular motion. Then rinse skin with tepid water. Afterward, pat skin dry. Skin will be moist and smooth. Use this scrub 2-3 times a week.

*Applying alpha hydroxy acid (AHA) or lactic acid-based creams *after* showering can provide gentle exfoliation and excellent skin hydration. A cost-effective, pH balanced AHA cream I personally use and recommend is **Evenly Radiant Overnight Peel**. Another one of my favorite hydrating and exfoliating body products is **Skinlasting Super Hydrator**. It's a powerful, yet gentle exfoliating mist that is formulated by a dermatologist. It's loaded with lactic acid which exfoliates and hydrates all skin types and contains green tea, vitamin C and hydrating hyaluronic acid. This unscented formulation keeps skin looking smooth, moist and firm for hours. Many women and men, including senior tennis players and golfers use this product to keep their legs and arms looking more youthful when wearing sleeveless tops and short tennis/golf skirts.

*Peptides can build collagen and increase the skin's hydration. After showering, apply a topical peptide-rich cream or serum. I recommend **Uplift Serum** which contains two types of peptides, skin firming DMAE, hyaluronic acid (HA) and antioxidants in a water base. Peptides are clinically documented to stimulate collagen over 350% and hydration over 260%. HA plumps and moisturizes, and antioxidants nourish and help repair the skin. For even more efficacy, I recommend massaging emu oil over Uplift Serum. Emu oil pushes the active peptides and skin firming antioxidant ingredients deep into the dermis where collagen forms. It also thickens skin and is 100% natural.

*Hyaluronic Acid (HA) holds 1000 times its weight in water. It quickly quenches dehydrated skin with loss of elasticity. The products noted above also contain HA. Another good choice is **Hydrating Hyaluronic Acid Mist.** Read more benefits of oral HA in **Age-Proofing Tip #51 - My Favorite Supplements for Women.**

*For thick skin buildup on knees, exfoliation is key. The easiest remedy is applying alpha hydroxy acid (AHA) moisturizer onto knees twice daily. AHAs naturally exfoliate, hydrate and soften all skin types. Apply it after showering in the morning and again at bedtime. I recommend cost-effective, pH balanced **Evenly Radiant Overnight Peel.**

*Make the following leg moisturizer that can help tighten skin. **Here's what you do:**

Melt one small ¾ oz. jar of shea butter in the microwave (without the lid). Break open 10 evening primrose oil capsules and add to the shea butter. Next add 10 drops lemongrass essential oil and 3 tbsp. emu oil and stir well. Allow to cool to room temperature. Apply and massage thighs. Lemongrass contains key skin-tightening properties.

*Skin rolling is a somewhat unheard of massage that has been around for over 20 years. It involves rolling and pinching of the skin to break up cellulite and fat deposits. In addition, it stimulates the skin and helps detoxify and sculpt the body. You'll be amazed at how much dead skin comes off the body during a skin rolling treatment.

*While watching TV, massage thighs and tummy using an electric massager or a rolling pin to help break down cellulite. You can also perform chopping strokes (hands in a karate-like position), moving up and down the fatty areas of the thighs and buttocks. Kneading the skin is also beneficial.

*Bentonite clay draws out impurities and helps tighten thigh skin. **Here's what to do:**

In a glass bowl combine ½ cup water or apple cider vinegar with ¾ cup bentonite or China clay. Stir to a paste consistency and apply to cellulite-prone areas. Let dry. You will feel a tightening or pulling sensation. Wash clay off in the shower with tepid water.

*My cellulite-reduction oil recipe can be massaged onto thighs and legs. **Here's what you do:**

Combine 10 tbsp. almond oil or olive oil, 4 tsp. emu oil, 16 drops fennel essential oil, 12 drops rosemary essential oil, 2 drops grapefruit seed extract (preservative) and massage this combination onto cellulite-prone each night before bed.

Camouflage Cellulite with Self-Tanner

Self-tanner can help camouflage cellulite on the legs. Some of the most famous lingerie models use self-tanner for this reason. Yes, even models battle cellulite. For legs, I recommend Vani-T® Bronzing Custard from Australia. It's free of parabens and phthalate-fragrances and it provides a sun-kissed, bronzy glow. In addition, the key ingredients include natural hydrating oils such as macadamia, sunflower and coconut, vitamins E and A, and it's scented with natural extracts such as sage and vanilla. Bronzing Custard is excellent for dry, winter skin and the scent is very mild, unlike many other self-tanners.

Applying self-tanner on legs is now far easier than ever before. **Here's what you do:**

Prior to application, exfoliate skin in the shower. To do this, pour some baking soda on a wet face cloth and gently scrub the legs in a circular motion. Dry brushing the legs prior to showering is another skin exfoliating option. Then shave legs. Self-tanner goes on more smoothly when legs are hairless. After showering, pat skin dry. Afterward, apply a nickel-sized amount of tanner and massage it in a circular motion from foot up to knee. Circular massage application prevents streaks. Next, massage a quarter-sized amount of tanner beginning from the upper knee to the top of the thigh. Repeat on other leg. Afterward, wash hands with soap and water. For a darker skin tone, re-apply every 48 hours until desired tone is achieved. To maintain the tone, re-apply once or twice weekly.

Also check out my natural self-tanner recipe below. It's made with black tea.

Make Your Own Self-Tanner (arms & legs)

Instead of sunbathing or using controversial tanning beds, my natural self-tanner recipe gives skin a healthy sun-kissed glow. It will not rub off onto clothes and will stay put provided you're not dancing, swimming or working up a sweat. I recommend this recipe for a non-dancing date, dinner out or party. It stays on until showered off. And it's healthy for skin too. Black tea provides a nice, non-orange shade as well as anti-inflammatory tannins. **Here's what you do:**

You will need 12 (black) tea bags for this recipe. Boil 1 cup water. Place 6 tea bags into the boiled water and let steep for 20 minutes. Remove the tea bags, making sure to squeeze each tea bag well. Re-boil the steeped tea water. Add 6 more tea bags to the re-boiled tea and steep again. Squeeze each tea bag well when removing them. Allow the tea water to cool to room temperature. To apply the self-tanner, dip a bristle-hair pastry brush into the tea mixture and 'paint' the tanner onto clean legs and arms using long, even strokes. Allow the tea to dry for 7-10 minutes before getting dressed.

Fade Spider Veins

Reddish-blue spider veins usually become more visible on the legs during hormonal stages and pregnancy. Below are some effective and affordable suggestions that can help reduce the look of these small, yet noticeable veins.

*Good circulation helps prevent spider veins. Uncross your legs when sitting and put feet up at the end of the day - especially if your job requires standing for long hours.

*Standing or sitting on a vibration plate provides tremendous circulation. Whether set on low or high speeds, this therapy can address spider veins, balance hormones, reduce cellulite, and more. Read about **Body Vibration Plates** in **Age-Proofing Tip #58.**

*Applying self-tanner can reduce the look of spider veins. See my self-tanner recipe above or try **Tan Toner** noted in **Age-Proofing Tip #34 - Camouflaging Vilitigo** or **Bronzing Custard**® noted earlier in this section.

*Oral supplements such as gingko biloba, grapeseed extract, butcher's broom extract, horse chestnut, vitamin C, bioflavonoids, beta carotene, vitamin E and zinc can improve circulation and strengthen veins. Many leg and vein oral formulations combine many of these supplements. Find them at health food stores.

*Clinical studies note that herbal horse-chestnut (tincture) improves leg circulation, decreases inflammation, and strengthens the capillaries and veins. Below is an effective recipe. **Here's what you do:**

Combine 3 tbsp. witch hazel with 1 tsp. horse chestnut (homeopathic tincture) and apply on spider veins. Then apply emu oil overtop and massage into the affected areas.

*Apply homeopathic arnica gel or cream and then massage emu oil overtop. Arnica helps fade bruising as well as reddish-blue spider veins. Emu oil will speed your results. Try this natural and safe combination for 90 days.

*An affordable and effective spider vein treatment is sclerotherapy. It's one of the fastest ways to reduce spider and small varicose veins. A solution is injected using an ultra-fine tipped needle which causes the veins to instantly collapse. Within two weeks the veins lighten in color. Do not exercise for at least one week after having this treatment. Seek an experienced vein specialist to prevent scarring. This procedure can be performed on hands too.

Victoria's Secret® Model Tips for Long, Leaner-Looking Legs

I've noted a few Victoria's Secret® model insider tips for longer-looking legs. In addition to applying self-tanner to camouflage cellulite, makeup artists apply highlighting foundation in a long strip (about one inch wide), down the front and back of the models legs. This highlighting 'strip' creates the illusion of longer, thinner legs. Many female celebrity guests on late night talk shows use this leg slimming illusion too.

Here's another model tip. Many Victoria's Secret® models reveal that they go on a liquid protein diet and eat veggies *only* approximately two weeks prior to their annual runway show to reduce cellulite and enhance muscle-tone.

An Affordable Cellulite & Body Contouring Treatment

Arasis® Inch Loss System is an effective and non-invasive body contouring and cellulite treatment that can tighten and restore elasticity in the connective tissue. It helps tone muscle too. This treatment was originally developed for those with multiple sclerosis yet proved so effective at tightening skin, that medical professionals now use the Arasis® system for various clinical purposes. It has been available in Europe since 2002, but is quite new to the USA. Aestheticians use it for inch loss and cellulite smoothing, gynecologists incorporate the treatment to tighten abdominal muscles after childbirth, and plastic surgeons use it to tighten skin after a liposuction. It is safe and non-invasive with zero side effects.

How does it work?

You may recall the muscle-toning devices from the past that used electrical currents to stimulate muscles. The Arasis® uses no direct electrical current; but, rather it targets the nerves that control the muscles. The wavelengths trigger a bio-electric signal from the brain to the body to create a deep muscle contraction, much like doing exercise. This affordable treatment is like a combination of micro-current and electronic muscle stimulation but goes far deeper for a faster result. The benefit of Arasis® is that the muscles don't feel sore after a treatment because it burns fat and tones without depleting glucose. Arasis® is combined with a pre-treatment called Vacuodermie® which targets cellulite, provides lymphatic drainage, improves body contours, eliminates toxins, and improves cellular regeneration. Muscle tone is improved, skin looks smoother and many report losing inches. This dual treatment takes about one hour and costs approximately $200 at Brentwood Medical Group and Laser Center. Mention Hollywood Beauty Secrets when you make an appointment and receive a free complimentary consultation and a discount. Watch for further price reductions on Groupon®. **NOTE:** Price noted is subject to change.

New York Leg Model's Secret Workout

A friend of mine is considered one of New York's top leg models. Though she's now over 45, she still has THE most amazing legs. She gave me permission to share her personal leg and butt workout. These exercises are very demanding due to the number of repetitions. With persistence you'll work up to the required reps which will result in tightened, sculpted, toned legs and buttocks. Perform the exercises in less than 20 minutes every other day. You can even do some of the exercises in the office while on the phone, or while watching TV. **Here's what you do:**

1. Press your back against the wall, in a sitting position (as if sitting on a chair). Hold this position until legs start shaking. Then hold for an additional count of 20 before coming out of the position. This exercise works thighs, hamstrings and butt.

2. While holding 3 lb. to 5 lb. weights in each hand, alternate 20 lunges on each leg until you've done three sets for a total of 60 reps per leg. This may seem like a lot, but truly worth the leg and butt-firming results.

3. While kneeling on all fours, lift and extend right leg back with foot flexed; lift leg up 20 times. Then lift the same leg out to the side 20 times. Switch legs and repeat. Do 3 sets of 20 on each leg.

4. While kneeling on all fours, lift right leg up, bend at the knee and flex foot up toward the ceiling. Keeping the foot flexed, lift leg up 20 times. Then repeat with other leg until you've done 3 sets on each leg. This workout is demanding 'butt' really works!

See more body toning exercises in **Age-Proofing Tip #57 - Weight Resistance Exercise.** Also check out *Body Vibration Plates* to help tone, lose inches, reduce cellulite and more in **Age-Proofing Tip #58.**

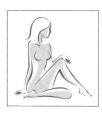

Age-Proofing Tip #46
Bath and Body

As noted at the beginning of my book, it is best to use paraben and phthalate-free products on the body to avoid hormone imbalances and other health issues. Below are some of my favorite natural body cleansers and soothing bath recipes for all skin types.

Paraben & Phthalate-Free Body Cleanser Choices

There are many body products available in health food stores across the country, though several still contain synthetic fragrances which are phthalates. Check with the manufacturer to be sure. If you like a scent, choose products that are <u>naturally</u> scented with essential oils. My favorite body washes are **Jason®** **Body Shower Gel** (aloe vera), economical **Everyone® Soap** and **Burt's Bees Peppermint & Rosemary Body Wash**. See more products noted in **Safe, Effective Face & Body Product Suggestions**.

Paraben & Phthalate-Free Deodorant Choices

A highly effective deodorant is **Aubrey® E Plus High C Roll-On Deodorant**. It surprisingly keeps both my husband and me dry, unlike other natural deodorants. Also the light, natural scent is fine for women, men or teens. Another nice men's choice is **Rock® Deodorant Spray** (onyx natural scent). These deodorants are healthy and help mask body odor.

<u>**Odor-reducing tip:**</u> One reason for sudden strong body odor may be a deficiency of zinc. Approximately 35% of women are low in zinc which can cause myriad issues including falling hair, depression, acne and body odor. A daily intake of 25 mg of zinc can help. Check with your health practitioner before taking supplements.

Soothing Bath Recipes

Indulge in any one of the following 10 soothing bath recipes whenever you have 30 minutes to relax. **NOTE:** Do not take baths with essential oils if pregnant as they penetrate into the skin very deeply.

*Coconut milk is rich in anti-microbial and yeast-fighting property caprylic acid. It also contains skin-hydrating oils that soothe dry skin. **Here's what you do:**

Add 1 can unsweetened coconut milk to a warm bath. Relax in the tub for 15 minutes. Do not rinse off. Simply pat skin dry.

*Japanese women have taken green tea baths for centuries. Green tea is rich in skin firming, hydrating and rejuvenating properties. It improves collagen production for firmer and more youthful-looking skin. In addition, green tea provides UV protection from the sun and anti-microbial properties that help keep blemishes in check. **Here's what you do:**

Steep 8 green tea bags in 2 cups water and add to tepid bath water. Relax in the tub for 15 minutes. Do not rinse skin. Simply pat skin dry.

*Milk is a wonderful exfoliating bath ingredient for all skin types including those with eczema or dry skin. It is rich in lactic acid to help gently exfoliate and even the skin tone. Also, the fat in milk moisturizes skin. Cold milk cools the bath water so make certain you run <u>hot</u> water for this bath recipe. **Here's what you do:**

Add 1 gallon whole milk to hot bath water. Relax in the bath for 20 minutes. Rinse with tepid water. You may substitute milk with 2 cups powdered milk.

*After a hectic day, my oatmeal and herb bath is very soothing. **Here's what you do:**

Sprinkle 4 tbsp. dry oatmeal, 5 dried sage leaves, 1 tbsp. dried rosemary and ¼ cup apple cider vinegar into tepid bath water. Relax in the bath for 20 minutes. Do not rinse skin. Simply pat skin dry.

*Apple cider vinegar relieves dry, itchy skin. **Here's what you do:**

Add 1 cup apple cider vinegar to a tub of tepid water. Soak for 20 minutes. Do not rinse skin. Simply pat skin dry.

*Experiencing stiff muscles or a sore back? **Here's what you do:**

Add 5 drops peppermint essential oil and 5 drops rosemary essential oil to bath water. Soak for 20 minutes. Do not rinse skin. Simply towel off.

*To increase circulation this bath recipe is very effective. **Here's what you do:**

Add 4 drops eucalyptus oil and 4 drops thyme essential oil to tepid bath water. Relax in the bath for 20 minutes. Then rinse and pat skin dry.

*For a soothing bath or for those with eczema, this is an excellent hydrating bath recipe. **Here's what you do:**

Steep 8 chamomile tea bags in 3 cups boiling water. Remove tea bags, and add tea to tepid tub water. Tannins in chamomile can help relieve inflammation, itching and dry skin. Relax in the bath for 20 minutes. Do not rinse skin. Simply pat skin dry.

*For detoxifying the body and reducing inflammation, Epsom® salts are beneficial. Key ingredient magnesium sulphate helps release toxins from the skin and can reduce foot swelling. **Here's what you do:**

Add 1 cup Epsom® salts and 2 tbsp. olive or jojoba oil into tepid bath water and soak for 20 minutes. Rinse and pat skin dry.

*My honey and lavender bath is soothing and calming. **Here's what you do:**

Add 4 tbsp. dried lavender, 1 cup whole milk, ¼ cup raw honey, and 2 tbsp. jojoba oil to tepid bath water. Relax in the bath for 20 minutes. Rinse and pat skin dry.

Bath Salt Recipes

My bath salt recipes can be used for relaxing or energizing. They make great gifts too. A relaxing bath salt recipe is something every woman can enjoy. **Here's what you do:**

To make a relaxing salt bath recipe, combine 1 cup Himalayan pink salt, ¼ cup almond or olive oil and 6 drops lavender essential oil. Mix well. Then add ¼ cup of the bath salts to tepid bath water and enjoy this relaxing bath. Store the remaining bath salts in a Glad® storage container.

When you need a pick-me-up, an energizing salt bath can do the trick. **Here's what you do:**

To make an energizing salt bath recipe, combine 1 cup Himalayan pink salt, ¼ cup almond or olive oil and 6 drops peppermint essential oil. Mix well. Then add ¼ cup of the bath salts to tepid bath water. Store the remaining bath salts in a Glad® storage container.

Body Moisturizers

*Skin is the body's largest organ which is why I recommend moisturizing with natural oils. **NOTE:** Natural oils can go rancid quickly so make body oil recipes in small batches and place unused oils in the refrigerator to keep them fresh until needed. After bathing or showering, apply oil on clean skin to seal in moisture. Below are some effective body moisturizing recipes.

*I love my body butter beautifier recipe. It's made with shea butter, coconut and safflower oil. Shea butter is moisturizing. Coconut oil is rich in fatty acids that reduce inflammation, help fade scars and hydrate all skin types. Safflower oil is rich in plant-based omega 6s. **Here's what you do:**

Melt ½ cup shea butter and ¼ cup coconut oil (food grade) in the microwave. Then add 3 tbsp. safflower oil and 1 tsp. vodka to the melted butter. Vodka is a natural preservative. If you don't have vodka, add 2 drops Nutribiotic® Grapefruit Seed Extract to the mixture. Smooth the butter on body and/or dry, cracked feet.

*This body moisturizer is a classic. It's fast and simple to make. **Here's what you do:**

Combine 1 cup almond or grape seed oil with 10 drops fragrant essential oil such as lavender or grapefruit.

See more body moisturizer recipes in **More Beauty Recipes** and find products in **Safe, Effective Face & Body Product Suggestions.**

Laser Hair Removal

Laser hair removal has come a long way over the years. It is the one of fastest growing, non-surgical treatments. Both women and men can use this treatment on all areas of the body. Best of all, it is now a more affordable and comfortable treatment than ever before. Effective ***Cynosure® Elite*** can be used on all skin and hair types. Cynosure® combines two wavelengths (755 and 1064 nm) which have been proven to offer optimal hair removal results. In addition, the laser is combined with SmartCool®, which is considered one of the best skin cooling methods and enhances comfort during each session. Usually 3-10 sessions are required depending on the area of treatment. Great deals on laser hair removal treatments are frequently listed at Groupon®.com. It's free to join so sign up for outstanding offers.

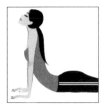

Age-Proofing Tip #47
Joint Support

One of my clients, a Hollywood set designer for many popular television shows, mentioned to me that he suffered from terrible knee pain and was scheduled for knee surgery. He asked if I had any suggestions so I recommended that he take hyaluronic acid (HA) supplements to help cushion the cartilage in his knees. Just one month later he was ecstatic. The HA supplement not only banished his knee pain, he cancelled his surgery! Read more benefits of HA below:

Hyaluronic acid (HA) is a substance that our bodies naturally produce. However, with age we slow down producing HA which can result in dry, aged-looking skin, poor vision and aching joints. As noted on earlier pages, applying topical HA on skin hydrates and plumps up wrinkles. HA quenches thirsty skin. Because of its high molecular weight, HA has the ability to bind to water. When taken as an oral supplement, HA hydrates skin from the inside out, lubricates the eyes, and stimulates the production of natural joint fluid which reduces sore, aching joints. When our joints lack proper lubrication, the bones rub together. Over time, this damages the spongy cartilage on the ends of bones. If you're like many Americans who experience painful, aching joints, you can experience incredible relief by taking oral hyaluronic acid. Other benefits of taking HA are improved eyesight and younger-looking skin. HA can help 'turn back the clock'. I've recommended HA to many of my clients, family and friends. They ALL reported that HA provided joint pain relief within <u>days</u>.

Astaxanthin® is a powerful rejuvenating antioxidant that fights free radicals. In addition, it provides a drug-free alternative for addressing the signs of aging, from chronic joint and muscle pain, to inflammation and wrinkles. With long term use Astaxanthin® can help reduce back pain, osteo and rheumatoid arthritis, carpal tunnel, tennis elbow, inflammation in joints, and sore muscles. Many professional athletes take oral Astaxanthin® supplements as part of their daily regimens to increase stamina and reduce post-workout inflammation. The added benefit of taking Astaxanthin® is that it's age-defying! It helps reduce wrinkles! Find it in foods such as salmon, shrimp, lobster and other foods rich in red color or take oral supplements.

Krill oil is derived from crustaceans found in the ocean and is a common food eaten by whales, penguins and seals. It is rich in omega 3 fatty acids and can protect cells from free radical damage. Krill supports the nervous system, brain function and can reduce bad LDL cholesterol. Fitness guru Johnathan Jones recommends krill oil as an effective joint support supplement. In addition, a study conducted by *Journal of the American College of Nutrition* examined krill oil and reported that taking 300 mg daily was effective at reducing arthritis symptoms and inflammation. **NOTE:** Do not take krill oil if allergic to shellfish, have bleeding concerns or if taking blood thinners including aspirin or ginkgo biloba, to name a few.

Hot peppers such as cayenne, habanero or jalapeno contain powerful circulatory phytochemicals. The key property of these peppers is capsaicin which aids blood flow to aching joints. Peppers are known to improve brain function and heart health, unblock the lymphatic system, maintain healthy blood pressure and even strengthen nerves, capillaries and arteries. If you have joint pain or circulation issues, talk to your doctor about cayenne, habanero or jalapeno peppers in capsule form. A popular natural formula that blends these powerful peppers is ***Dr. Schulze Cayenne Powder Blend***. Get more information and order it online at HerbDoc.com.

Pomegranates are one of the most potent antioxidant fruits. They help maintain healthy cells, and can help reduce joint inflammation. Other foods reported to help calm joint pain are ***bazil nuts, sunflower*** and ***pumpkin seeds***.

Ginger is a powerful, natural remedy that is known to help calm stiff joints and muscle soreness. It contains an enzyme that blocks inflammation. Use it as a spice for cooking or making ginger tea.

Since our bodies do not store ***vitamin C***, a daily supplement and eating vitamin C-rich foods are recommended to protect joints and stimulate collagen production within bone cartilage. Osteoarthritis and joint pain may be a result of chronic inflammation due to the breakdown of cartilage. According to a study performed at *Boston University*, a minimum of 150 mg of vitamin C daily is recommended to prevent cartilage deterioration. Also consider taking Pycnogenol®, an antioxidant that is 20 times more effective than vitamin C. Read more about age-defying Pycnogenol® in **Age-Proofing Tip #51 - My Favorite Supplements for Women**.

Vitamin D can support healthy joint cartilage. Vitamin D is available in supplement form and found in foods such as milk, fatty fish and liver. Read many more benefits of vitamin D in **Age-Proofing Tip #51 - My Favorite Supplements for Women**.

Trans-resveratrol is a powerful phyto nutrient found in grape seeds, skins, and a root called knotweed. Trans-resveratrol is the most potent form of resveratrol. It can contribute to our overall health and wellbeing. *Harvard* researchers and countless other studies reveal that resveratrol contains anti-inflammatory agents that reduce pain, improve joint health and support cartilage, increase energy, and help us look and feel younger. Though we've heard the buzz about red grape skins and seeds, it is knotweed that contains even <u>more</u> powerful trans-resveratrol. It is perfectly safe and has no known side effects - even at higher doses. Look for knotweed on labels. Read more about trans-resveratrol in **Age-Proofing Tip #56 - Boost Your Metabolism**.

Avoid foods that cause inflammation. According to a Canadian homeopathic expert, foods that can cause inflammation include peanuts, white potatoes, tomatoes, citrus fruits, dairy, red meat, and eggplant to name a few.

NOTE: As noted in the disclaimer, check with a healthcare professional before taking supplements.

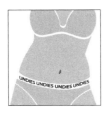

Age-Proofing Tip #48
Relieve Constipation, Bloating & Gas

Constipation causes bloating, gas, discomfort, hinders weight loss goals, affects energy and our outlook on life. Eight out of 10 women experience constipation which causes the colon to swell and affects the function of our other organs such as kidneys, liver, gallbladder, pancreas, uterus, adrenals and more. Our internal organs require good circulation to function at maximum efficacy.

"The average American stores from 10 to 12 pounds of fecal matter in his or her colon." – American Botanical Pharmacy

*If eating sufficient fiber, yet still experiencing constipation and bloating, try increasing your water intake from eight glasses a day to 10-12. In addition, incorporate the following effective relaxation ritual that can help induce a morning bowel movement without the use of laxatives.

FACT: A proper bowel movement takes about 10-15 minutes, allowing the muscles to relax. Many of us do not allow sufficient time 'to go'. A biokinesiologist in Pasadena introduced me to this highly effective stomach breathing exercise that can induce regular bowel movements. The combination of deep breathing and drinking water helps relax and hydrate the intestines. Within a few minutes, bowels will move with ease. **Here's what you do:**

Each morning, before rising from bed, close your eyes and place both hands on your stomach. Then count to five as you inhale S L O W L Y through your nose and into the abdomen. (Counting to five helps you to focus on relaxing). As you breathe in, the abdomen fills with air. Next, count to five as you breathe out (through your nose) while pulling the abdomen in (deflating the stomach). Repeat 20 times and be sure to breathe slowly to induce relaxation of the intestines and muscles. Then rise from bed and drink two to three glasses of room temperature water.

Fiber Facts You Need to Know

*Fiber stabilizes blood sugar levels, keeping the metabolism strong and disease free. In addition, consuming fiber can reduce blood pressure, enhance weight loss and prevent certain cancers. Over 200 studies have noted that consuming five to nine servings of high fiber fruits and vegetables can lower the risk of breast cancer development by 50% and colon cancer by 34%. In one breast cancer study, survivors with higher estrogen levels increased their fiber intake and experienced a significant

reduction in those levels. Additional studies note that a diet rich in fiber can prevent constipation and diseases such as ovarian and rectal cancer.

*When increasing fiber many individuals experience uncomfortable gas and bloating. It is recommended to slowly incorporate fiber into the diet - allowing up to 30 days for the body to adapt. **NOTE:** It is perfectly natural for gas and bloating to occur for up to one month, but will subside once the body adjusts. Increase fiber consumption by 10 grams per week until reaching 35.

*Be sure to drink more water (10-12 glasses a day) when incorporating more fiber-rich foods into your diet. Set a timer to sound off every hour as a reminder to drink a glass of water. It's amazing how quickly the hours can go by without drinking sufficient water - especially while at work.

*If dealing with constipation, hormonal imbalances, weight issues, diabetes or you want to look and feel better or younger, the following disease-fighting and fiber-rich foods and remedies can help. They provide post-meal satisfaction, reduce cravings for sweets, balance hormones, uplift our mood, reduce bloating and aid in weight loss.

High Fiber Foods & Supplements

Besides being high in fiber and low in calories, eating whole fruits and veggies provide antioxidant-rich, age-defying properties as well as protection from harmful UV rays. Be sure to eat fruit skins for additional fiber and avoid drinking fruit juices. They are high-glycemic, high in calories and provide very little fiber.

Flaxseeds
Rich in fiber and plant-based essential omega-3 fatty acids, flaxseeds are known to help balance and reduce levels of hormones linked to breast cancer. Flax ignites fat burning, uplifts our mood, supports heart health and provides relief of constipation and inflammation. Those with serious conditions such as painful arthritis and lupus report much relief when they incorporate flaxseed oil into their daily regimen. To help with constipation relief, grind flaxseeds and sprinkle them on yogurt, oatmeal, or fruit; in a protein smoothie, bran muffin or pancake recipe. Add flaxseed oil to salad dressing or mix it into tuna salad. See my delicious high fiber, low carbohydrate pancake recipe in **My Favorite Healthy Meal & Snack Recipes**. Take flaxseed at bedtime too. **Here's what you do:**

Add 1 tbsp. flaxseed to 12 oz. room temperature water. Stir well and drink. Follow with another glass of water.

Yogurt and Probiotics

Yogurt provides millions of beneficial bacteria that can aid digestive issues, boost the immune system, uplift our mood, protect against cancer and induce a better bowel movement. Choose yogurt with labels that note live or active cultures and avoid those with sugar, corn syrup, or artificial sweeteners. Try plain Greek yogurt (more protein than others) and add low-glycemic berries, crushed walnuts, 1 tsp. of ground flaxseed, 1 tsp. raw sunflower seeds, or slivered almonds, and a little drizzle of honey on top. Low-glycemic berries include blueberries, raspberries, blackberries and strawberries. Plain, low-fat yogurt makes an excellent, creamy base for salad dressings and dips. For those experiencing a yeast infection or taking antibiotics (which can cause constipation), consider taking a daily probiotic to help support the digestive system. Read more about probiotics in **Age-Proofing Tip #51 - My Favorite Supplements for Women.**

Black Beans

I'm a huge fan of black beans. They are rich in fiber, highest in protein and low in calories. A half cup of black beans provides eight grams of protein and fiber. They're loaded with antioxidants that can help boost brain power and support heart health. Plus, they're free of saturated fat. Serve warm black beans with eggs for breakfast. They can be added to a breakfast wrap with eggs, avocado and cheese, in salads, chili and healthy tacos. Lentils, pinto beans, and peas are also rich in fiber. **TIP:** When eating red meat, eat a side dish of beans to help with elimination. Beef is harder to digest than other types of protein.

Garlic

According to an article published by *American Botanical Pharmacy*, there are at least 100 types of parasites that can enter our bodies via contaminated water, foods and the environment. In addition, a diet that is rich in sugar can cause bloating and an overgrowth of yeast. Garlic can help remedy bloating, bacteria, yeast and disease. It is rich in allicin, a key property that helps keep the entire system free of harmful microbes. Yeast overgrowth may be sabotaging your weight loss goals. Check with your doctor before taking a garlic supplement, especially if taking blood-thinning medications or have other health concerns.

Chlorella

Incredible, rejuvenating chlorella is a super toxinfighter and immune-booster that offers many health and beauty benefits. Because it is rich in detoxifying chlorophyll, chlorella can support the digestive system, induce bowel movements, balance hormones, freshen breath and purify the bloodstream and liver. Take 15 chlorella pellets first thing in the morning with a glass of water and then 10-15 pellets with lunch and dinner to help remedy constipation. Read even more benefits of chlorella in **Age-Proofing Tip #51 - My Favorite Supplements for Women.**

Habanero Peppers

According to leading herbalist Dr. Schulze at *American Botanical Pharmacy* in Los Angeles, habanero peppers can help stimulate muscular contractions that promote regular bowel movements.

Magnesium

Taking a magnesium supplement at bedtime can help loosen bowels by morning. It calms muscles inducing relaxation, reduces restless, twitching legs, and constipation. It is found in dairy products, pumpkin seeds, spinach, swiss chard, sunflower, and sesame seeds. In addition, magnesium helps relieve water retention and reduces pain associated with fibromyalgia, migraine headaches, muscle and joint pain, and chronic fatigue. **NOTE:** If taking thyroid or bone medications or antibiotics, check with your physician for the best time to take magnesium. Find magnesium supplements combined with calcium citrate at health food stores.

Psyllium Husk

Another effective, natural and cost-effective bedtime remedy is psyllium husk. Natural sources of psyllium are free of starch, sugar, salt, yeast, wheat, corn, milk, preservatives or color. **Here's what you do:**

Add 1 tbsp. ground psyllium to a 12 oz. glass of room temperature water. Stir well and quickly drink the mixture as it thickens immediately. Follow with another full glass of water.

Banish Bloating and Gas

*Avoid consuming bread and starches as they cause water retention and bloating. Choose quinoa instead of pasta or rice. Quinoa is rich in protein and fiber and is low-glycemic. Shiritaki noodles are another pasta alternative. They are high in fiber and virtually free of carbohydrates. My husband and I love these versatile noodles. See one of my favorite shiritaki recipes in **My Favorite Healthy Meal and Snack Recipes.**

*Avoid salt and diet sodas that contain sodium.

*Drink eight to ten glasses of water a day to prevent bloating. I increased my water intake for three days, lost three pounds, and my tummy flattened.

*Chewing on fennel seeds after a meal can help banish bad breath and eliminate gas or bloating. Swallow or discard seeds after chewing.

*Teas such as green, chamomile, mint, ginkgo, and cat's claw can help remedy bloating and stimulate circulation. In addition, green tea helps metabolize fat.

*Corn silk, made from fine strands of corn husk, is known for its many health benefits. It is a diuretic that reduces water retention, bloating and many other inflammatory conditions such as irritated urinary tract and bladder infections. Check with your doctor for its many uses including gout, kidney stones, prostate inflammation, diabetes, and much more. Be sure to choose a corn silk brand that was not sprayed with pesticides.

Improved Liver Function reduces bloating, gas, weight, IBS and more

The liver is one of our largest digestive glands. It filters everything we consume - including vitamins, medications and foods. In addition, the liver produces bile which is the key to breaking down, digesting and eliminating foods and fats. Improved bile production can eliminate bloating, constipation, hemorrhoids, cramping or gas, IBS, diarrhea, acid reflux, weight gain and other digestive challenges. Up to 70 million Americans are challenged with these symptoms. If you've tried probiotics, laxatives, antacids and colon cleansers and have experienced little relief, increasing the liver's bile production may help address the digestive issues noted above.

Author and British physician Dr. Scott-Mumby has published several books on nutrition and allergies. He also notes that bile, produced by the liver, plays a key role in digestion. Natural extracts derived from roots and plants including black radish root, artichoke, peppermint, and wormwood can stimulate bile, banish parasites, and improve many digestive and elimination challenges. Review the highlights of each natural ingredient below. Find them in combined in popular supplement **Dyflogest**™. The key ingredients include:

-black radish root - a powerful extract that triggers the liver to produce more bile. Bile improves and strengthens the liver and intestines. It also stimulates the muscular action in the intestines and colon to help with elimination;
-artichoke extract - stimulates the flow of bile from the liver to reduce heartburn symptoms and reduce the effects of IBS;

-<u>peppermint extract</u> - reduces nausea, diarrhea, gas and upset tummy; and

-<u>wormwood extract</u> - attacks harmful bacteria and parasites (hook and pinworms) and helps support liver, spleen, gallbladder, and kidney health.

Take Dyflogest™2 tablets in the morning and 2 at night or before consuming foods such as cabbage and beans. If you have a serious medical condition, please consult a physician before taking this supplement. **NOTE:** As noted earlier, use this product at your own risk. I was not paid to promote this or other products noted throughout these pages.

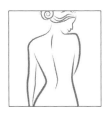

Age-Proofing Tip #49
Vaginal Balance

NOTE: Because there are several types of yeast infections, it is recommended that you consult a physician if you suspect an infection.

FACT: *Nearly 50% of women will experience a yeast infection twice in their lifetime.*

Healthy, balanced vaginal bacteria and flora can prevent the overgrowth of yeast. Yeast infections can be triggered by consuming sugary foods, taking contraceptives such as the pill, or antibiotics to treat other infections. Other causes of yeast overgrowth are stress or hormonal changes such as pregnancy, menstruation, menopause, and diabetes.

Signs of a yeast infection include:
-burning feeling during urination;
-pain, vaginal dryness or discomfort during intercourse;
-vaginal itching or tenderness; and
-thick vaginal discharge with an unpleasant odor.

A yeast infection can be prevented by:
-incorporating a balanced diet that includes pesticide-free vegetables, low-glycemic fruits, whole grains, low-fat dairy products, and reducing sugary foods or drinks;
-wearing cotton underwear and removing sweaty workout clothes immediately after exercise;
-eating yogurt and taking a daily probiotic especially when taking antibiotic medicines; and
-boosting the immune system with homeopathic vaginal formulations.

*To help reduce exterior vaginal itching and tenderness, apply coconut oil on clean skin nightly. Because it contains both lauric and caprylic acid, this antimicrobial blend can address yeast and topical fungal infections. When taken internally, coconut oil's caprylic acid is a natural yeast killer and does not affect good bacteria in the intestines. Women who consume coconut oil have a lower incidence of yeast infections. Apply coconut oil when challenged with vaginal itching and burning. **Here's what you do:**

Combine 1 tsp. coconut oil with 2 drops squalane oil (from olives) or emu oil and apply on clean skin twice daily. Be sure to see a health care professional if itching lasts more than a day or two.

*Homeopathic vaginal suppositories and gels can help trigger the body's natural ability to restore healthy flora without disrupting the protective bacteria. They are fine for those going through hormonal changes and vaginal dryness. These natural remedies can also address the treatment of bacterial vaginosis (BV) by restoring vaginal balance, and can provide speedy, gentle relief from burning or vaginal discharge. Choose homeopathic formulations that offer minerals, herbs, probiotics and other natural ingredients to help balance and fight existing yeast overgrowth conditions. An excellent brand of vaginal suppositories is **YeastGuard® Advanced Homeopathic Formulas**, a natural alternative to over-the-counter anti-fungal treatments. The suppositories are blended with probiotics, manufactured in compliance with FDA regulations and prepared under the *Homeopathic Pharmacopeia of the United States* (HPUS) guidelines. Find them at select drug and health food stores. **VH Essentials** is another homeopathic brand available at select drug stores.

*For temporary vaginal itching or yeast infection relief, prepare this effective douche recipe. **Here's what you do:**

Break open a probiotic capsule and stir into 1 cup warm distilled water. Do not use tap water. Douche with this mixture once a day for two days or until you can see your doctor.

*Another excellent yeast fighter is my doctor-recommended slimming tonic made with apple cider vinegar and garlic, noted in **Age-Proofing Tip #56 - Boost Your Metabolism.** Drink it first thing in the morning to help remedy an existing yeast infection or as a preventative when taking antibiotics.

Natural Personal Lubricant Alternative

Many personal lubricants can sting especially if skin is tender or inflamed due to vaginal itching. In addition, some commercial brands are sticky or contain fragrances (phthalates) and parabens. Many women going through hormonal changes experience vaginal dryness and sensitivity that makes intercourse uncomfortable and sometimes even painful. A healthy and effective vaginal lubricant is natural squalane oil derived from olives. Squalane is gentle and does not sting irritated skin. It is free of parabens, perfumes or phthalates and is hydrating, long lasting and never becomes sticky. It's the ultimate natural moisturizer for the delicate vaginal area both inside and out.

Age-Proofing Tip #50
Systemic Enzymes & Fibroids

Enzymes are catalysts that ignite all chemical reactions within the body. You've most likely heard of digestive enzymes which break down proteins, fats and starches in our food. Systemic enzymes are different in that they are taken orally on an empty stomach, and work within the bloodstream to positively impact our health in many ways - from turning back the clock to reducing pain, dissolving fibroids, arterial plaque and much more. Though many individuals are not familiar with these powerhouse enzymes, they have a forty-year history of widespread medical use in central Europe and Japan.

Systemic enzymes can effectively break down and 'digest' harmful proteins such as viruses and parasites, and excess scar tissue such as fibroids and keloids. They help eliminate toxins from the blood, liver and GI tract to support the immune system, and can play a role in reducing pain and inflammation. They even help slow aging. See even more benefits below.

There are currently over 200 peer-reviewed research articles dealing with the absorption and use of orally-administered systemic enzymes.

Quality Systemic Enzymes We Can Afford

Quality systemic enzyme formulations are usually prescribed by specialists and homeopathic practitioners. They are not readily available and are very costly. Recently my colleague, wellness expert, Stuart Spangenberg, introduced me to **Zymessence**™. This affordable systemic enzyme is formulated by William Wong, ND, Ph.D - a former spokesperson for another popular, but very costly, systemic enzyme formulation. Dr. Wong recognized that the high price of enzyme formulas made them inaccessible to those who would benefit from the therapy. After teaming up with a German pharmacologist, Zymessense™ was born. Dr. Wong's formulation is not only far more potent than many other brands, it is affordable. As you know, I uncover some of the most potent health and beauty products on the planet so I am very pleased to introduce you to Zymessense™.

Dr. Wong's digestive enzyme formulation is very potent, therefore you require fewer capsules. Other brands require taking <u>large</u> numbers of capsules three times a day. Many individuals report that taking only <u>one caplet</u> three times per day of Dr.

Wong's systemic enzymes, provide great results at a cost of just $1.50 per day! Below is a long list of health benefits of these powerhouse systemic enzymes. They can:

-slow the rate of aging by controlling inflammation;
-reduce arterial plaque;
-support the immune system;
-offer a safe alternative to non-steroidal anti-inflammatory drugs, such as aspirin and ibuprofen in controlling pain and inflammation;
-soften and reduce surgical scars;
-control inflammation and scarring after cosmetic surgery procedures;
-control fibrosis;
-dissolve uterine fibroid tumors, scar tissue, keloids, blood clots and cysts;
-open circulation by dissolving fibrin plugs in capillaries;
-dissolve endometrial tissue (painful endometriosis);
-dramatically improve fibrocystic breast symptoms;
-dissolve painful scar tissue that encapsulates breast implants;
-reduce joint pain and increase mobility;
-help the body repair damaged tissue and speed healing after an injury or surgery;
-improve most autoimmune conditions such as psoriasis, eczema, rosacea, lupus, MS, rheumatoid arthritis, Crohn's disease, and more;
-cleanse the blood, detoxify the colon, liver and promote better circulation;
-help quickly relieve herpes breakouts; and
-increase the efficacy other vitamins and food supplements.

NOTE: This product is not suitable for vegans or vegetarians. Choose **Vitalzyme X** instead. For more information about fibroid shrinkage, visit ShrinkFibroidsFast.com.

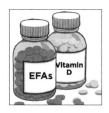

Age-Proofing Tip #51
My Favorite Supplements for Women

On earlier pages, I revealed many supplements that can help uplift our mood, enhance brain and organ function, support the immune system, induce relaxation, balance hormones, ignite fat burning and help reduce the risk of some cancers. A recent study revealed that taking vitamins has been proven to reduce the development of cancer by 40%. In addition to protecting us from free radicals, they can improve the look of our skin, and how we feel. I've highlighted some very powerful age-proofing supplements below.

NOTE: As noted in the disclaimer, check with your healthcare practitioner before trying new supplements.

__Plant-based__ omega 3 fatty acids are found in seeds, nuts and oils. They provide myriad health benefits that help reduce inflammation and turn back the clock. Our bodies require healthy fats for optimum skin and overall health. Omega 3 fatty acids can prevent dry, scaly skin, calm painful inflammation, help balance hormones, nourish the hair and nails, ignite fat-burning, uplift our mood, and calm anxiety and anger. A deficiency of omega 3 fatty acids can result in moodiness, thinning, dry, itchy and aged-looking skin, brittle nails, and dry or thinning hair. Our bodies cannot produce omega 3 fatty acids so we must get them from food sources. I recommend omega 3 sources that include flaxseeds and oil, evening primrose oil, walnuts, almonds, macadamia nuts and fresh fish such as wild salmon, trout and mackerel. I have been writing about the benefits of omega 3 fish oils for many years. However, I discovered some research back in 2011 that revealed some alarming news about fish oil supplements. Please read the new updates and warnings about fish oil below.

New Update & Warnings about Fish Oil Supplements

Many studies, including one from *Yale University* researchers and *Second Opinion's* alternative health physician, Dr. R. Rowen, uncovered some startling facts about fish oil. In early 2010, it was discovered that many fish oil supplements were tainted with mercury and other toxins (prior to packaging). While several others, when exposed to oxygen or heat, became rancid. Ingesting rancid fish oil triggers many serious health issues - blood clots, high insulin levels, weight gain, sore joints and inflammation. Inflammation causes us to age faster and look older too!

In addition, omega 3 fish oil supplements are high in unsaturated fat and <u>not</u> easily absorbed by the body. By taking fish oil in the amounts noted on most supplement bottles, many women and men have experienced a weight gain of 10 or more pounds as well as cravings for simple carbohydrates such as breads and sweets. In addition, many individuals report that they feel 'blue', look older than their years, and have been experiencing joint pain. Rancid fish oil may be the reason. Have you gained weight? Do you constantly crave carbs? The experts recommend switching to plant-based omega 3s such as those found in flax-seeds, flax oil, walnuts, leafy greens or <u>fresh</u> fish. Plant-based omega 3s are more easily absorbed by the body than fish oil. They retain their integrity in supplement form therefore chances of going rancid are slim. Nevertheless, I keep my plant-based omega 3s in the refrigerator to ensure that they stay fresh.

*In recent studies, ***<u>plant-based omega 6s</u>*** were found to be better for our health. Both plant-based omega 6s and omega 3s are much easier for the body to absorb and provide many health benefits when taken together. They help prevent spikes in blood sugar, uplift our mood, reduce inflammation, slow aging, reduce age spots, prevent artery stiffness, soothe stiff joints, support the immune system, balance hormones and insulin levels, reduce cholesterol and can help ignite fat-burning. **NOTE:** Do not confuse plant-based omega 6s with those found in processed foods. Those omega 6s are trans-fats (bad fats) that cause inflammation! Healthy omega 6 fatty acids are found in unprocessed oils such as evening primrose, borage, coconut, rice bran, sunflower and safflower oil. Healthy foods that are rich in omega 6s include beans, eggs, brazil nuts, almonds, cashews, sunflower and pumpkin seeds, and unsweetened coconut. So are plant-based omega 3s and 6s better than fish oil? Discuss these findings with your healthcare practitioner.

*Did you know that nearly ALL overweight women have LOW levels of ***vitamin D3*** and women who take higher levels of vitamin D3 experience 80% less abdominal fat? Vitamin D helps break down fat in the liver, it reduces food cravings, prevents depression, uplifts mood, increases energy, reduces eczema and psoriasis, halts throbbing or migraine headaches, improves bone density, aids immune function and production of healthy cells, reduces the risk of breast and colon cancer 30-50%, and maintains a strong immune system. According to a research at *McGill University*, vitamin D can help stop cancer. Their research reveals that vitamin D blocks the protein c-MYC, which is responsible for the cell division in more than 50% of ALL cancers. Additional studies note that vitamin D3 may help prevent a heart attack, can calm asthma and rheumatoid arthritis, keep blemishes in check and help the body absorb calcium. Find vitamin D in eggs, milk, cod, wild salmon, shrimp, liver and other organ meats. Almost all women are deficient in vitamin D3, especially those challenged with obesity issues because it is a fat soluble supplement. Have your vitamin D levels checked. It's an affordable blood test.

Chlorella is a nutrient-packed freshwater green algae, rich in healing vital nutrients and age-defying nucleic acid that helps reduce wrinkles, dry skin, adult acne, and enhances hair and nail growth. In addition, this powerhouse algae helps balance hormones, freshen breath, and prevent constipation. Chlorella is a super toxin fighter and immune booster that can turn back the clock. I revealed chlorella in my first book, *"Hollywood Beauty Secrets: Remedies to the Rescue,"* written in 2002. To date, it is still at the top of my list as one of the best nutritional supplements on the planet. Chlorella contains 19 essential amino acids that can help boost immunity. It contains more pantothenic acid (B5) than any other source. It is rich in chlorophyll, a powerful detoxifying property that can help clean the liver and bloodstream and can even bind to heavy metals to help safely remove them from the system. It even binds to mercury! How chlorella is processed is the key to getting the most potent quality. Some manufacturers use methods such as bleaching or heat-freezing which can destroy the nutrients. Others smash the cell walls, harming the nutrients.

Choose chlorella that is not grown in open ponds to avoid pesticides, fertilizers and environmental toxins. Those toxins bind to chlorella, and when consumed, our bodies absorb them! One brand I like is King Chlorella. It is made with filtered water, no fertilizers or pesticides, and harvests are strictly monitored and tested. Added probiotics in this brand also help protect the immune system. Take 10 - 15 pellets prior to bedtime or after each meal of the day.

Hyaluronic acid (HA) is a substance that our bodies produce naturally. It is present in the upper layers of our skin (dermis), in our eyes, and cushions our joints. As we age, our natural production of HA slows down. However, when applied topically or taken as an oral supplement, HA is truly age-defying. I noted on earlier pages that topical applications of HA can boost the skin's elasticity and hydration. It instantly plumps up wrinkles, quenches thirsty skin, enhances and firms the skin tone and cushions collagen. When taken as an oral supplement, HA plumps the skin and boosts hydration and elasticity from the inside out. In addition, taking HA supplements lubricate the eyes and calm sore, aching joints by cushioning the cartilage. HA lubricates the spongy cartilage on the ends of our bones which halts joint pain. Several individuals that I have recommended this supplement to report joint pain relief within DAYS! Taking HA supplements can improve eyesight, possibly reducing the need for reading glasses. For those with sun-damaged or wrinkled skin, dry eyes, or sore joints, taking oral HA supplements are most beneficial. Read more about HA in **Age-Proofing Tip #39 - Brighter Youthful-Looking Eyes.**

*I have sung the praises of powerful antioxidant, **Pycnogenol**®, for over 10 years. It is a natural extract derived from French maritime pine that is proven to be 50 times more powerful than vitamin E and 20 times more powerful than vitamin C. It can be applied topically or taken as an oral supplement. When applied topically, Pycnogenol® can neutralize free radicals to help prevent and reverse the visible signs of aging such as dehydration and wrinkles. In addition, it calms inflammatory skin conditions such as rosacea and broken capillaries. When taken as an oral supplement, it can fade melasma and age spots from the inside out. Those challenged with inflammation associated with irritable bowel syndrome, digestive issues or joint pain can benefit from Pycnogenol® as well. It reduces swelling, improves circulation and increases blood flow to help the body naturally heal itself. Pycnogenol® is an antioxidant has no known side effects. Find oral supplement at all health food stores. A powerful topical skin care formulation I've recommended for the past decade is **Age-defying Night Crème.** It is an advanced concentration that combines both Pycnogenol® and Astaxanthin® (another powerhouse antioxidant) and is free of paraben, phthalates, petroleum or synthetic colors. Find it in **Safe, Effective Face & Body Product Suggestions.**

***Astaxanthin*®** is a super antioxidant that can neutralize a variety of free radicals making it one of THE ultimate antioxidants. When applied topically, Astaxanthin® is age-defying! It reduces lines and wrinkles and helps repair, nourish and protect the skin. When taken as an oral supplement, it strengthens the cells (inside and out) and protects the organs, skin, eyes, and joints. Astaxanthin® reduces swelling associated with chronic joint and back pain, osteo and rheumatoid arthritis, carpal tunnel, tennis elbow, and sore muscles. Many professional athletes incorporate Astaxanthin® as part of their daily regimen to increase stamina and reduce post-workout inflammation. It is also found in many foods including salmon, shrimp, lobster and other foods rich in red color.

*Krill oil is rich in omega 3 fatty acids, protects cells from free radical damage, can help support the nervous system, brain function, and can reduce bad LDL cholesterol. A study conducted by the *Journal of the American College of Nutrition* recommends 300 mg daily in order to reduce arthritis symptoms and joint pain. Read more about the anti-inflammatory and joint pain relief of krill oil in **Age-Proofing Tip #47 - Joint Support. NOTE:** Krill oil is derived from crustaceans found in the ocean. Do not take krill oil if allergic to shell fish, have bleeding concerns or taking blood thinners including aspirin or ginkgo biloba, to name a few. **FYI:** My mom has suffered for several years with severe joint pain in her knees and hips (osteoarthritis). When I suggested that she stop taking fish oil and incorporate oral hyaluronic acid, krill oil and Astaxanthin® - her joint pain stopped - within DAYS. She is now pain free. I've been shouting this from the rooftops. The supplement I recommended combined all three supplements. It's called Joint Care by Schiff®.

*Fat-soluble *vitamin K2* can protect against bone loss and osteoporosis. K2's main job is to transport calcium from the bloodstream to the bones to enhance bone density. In addition, K2 prevents calcium from forming in the arteries which can prevent cardiovascular blockages (clogged arteries). Lower bone mineral density indicates a deficiency of vitamin K2. One study concluded that those low in vitamin K are more likely to experience a hip fracture. A Japanese study noted that K2 may decrease the risk of liver cancer by 20%. Foods rich in vitamin K are kale, brussel sprouts, spinach and green beans. It can help keep the arteries clear too.

*Magnesium not only helps uplift us, it prevents mood swings, relieves water retention, protects bones, nerves and muscle, and reduces migraine and fibromyalgia pain. Taking a magnesium supplement at bedtime calms muscles, restless legs or twitching, induces relaxation and halts bruxism (grinding teeth while sleeping). Grinding teeth is a sign of stress. In addition, taking magnesium at bedtime helps loosen bowels by morning so can be helpful to those challenged with constipation. Find magnesium in dairy products and foods such as pumpkin seeds, spinach, swiss chard and sunflower seeds. **NOTE:** Magnesium can interfere with some medications so check with your doctor on the best time to take it.

*Pantothenic acid (**vitamin B5**) is an excellent supplement that addresses adrenal support. It can help uplift the mood, prevent irritability and depression, and is a key supplement for those going through all stages of menopause. Vitamin B5 helps the body convert food to energy. For those with low energy, or a hectic schedule, consider taking pantothenic acid daily. Find it in eggs, bananas, beans, avocados, broccoli, and nuts.

***Folic acid, B6 and B12,** often found in multivitamins, can assist memory function, protect the nervous system, help fight infection and protect DNA. Find them in eggs, meat, liver, seafood, fruits, nuts, vegetables, avocados, whole grains and beans. Garbanzo beans, spinach and broccoli are high in folic acid and recommended for those who are feeling 'blue.'

***Green tea** offers myriad age-proofing and health benefits. It contains anti-inflammatory agents that fight free radicals and prevent loss of glutathione (a natural detoxifier found in every cell of the body), which protects our health. More benefits of green tea include improved collagen production for firm, more youthful-looking and hydrated skin, UV protection from the sun, and anti-microbial properties that help keep blemishes in check. It boosts memory power, enhances joint mobility, stabilizes blood sugar levels, and stimulates fat burning, speeds weight loss and more. A study performed at the *Western University of Health Sciences* revealed that drinking green tea can lower 'bad' LDL cholesterol and triglycerides. Another study published in *Nutrition Research* noted that green tea (in the form of an extract) can reduce blood pressure, diabetes, insulin resistance and heart disease. Drinking a cup of green tea both before AND after each meal of the day is known to speed weight loss. Some individuals report dropping up to 15 pounds per year. The key thermogenic property is EGCG (epigallocatechin) a catechin that induces fat burning and protects us from free radicals. If you're not a fan of drinking green tea, try **Thermo Green Tea**™ extract in capsule form. It offers a precise ratio of EGCG proven to increase thermogenesis by up to 43%, will not increase heart rate or cause jitters and is ephedra-free. I take it myself when I want to enhance my weight loss goals. You can bathe in green tea too. Japanese women have used this skin rejuvenating bath for centuries.

*Taking a combination of **vitamin B6, evening primrose oil** and **vitamin E** before menstruation can help relieve symptoms of PMS-related depression, tender breasts and the inflammation that flares up during this time of the month.

*Taking 1000 mg of **vitamin C** or **fat-soluble C-ester** daily is recommended by anti-aging experts. Vitamin C is a powerful antioxidant that can help reduce the development of heart disease, support our immune system and capillaries, and combat inflammation to help slow aging, prevent pain and other diseases. Find vitamin C in citrus fruits and vegetables.

*CoQ10 is a powerful, fat-soluble antioxidant that supports every cell in the body. It boosts our memory, energy, strengthens the heart, addresses diabetes, enhances weight loss and calms pain. Several studies note that CoQ10 can help relieve the stiffness associated with Parkinson's disease and calms fibromyalgia pain and migraine headaches. By age 35, the body begins producing less CoQ10 so taking a daily supplement supports the heart, increases energy, uplifts mood and enhances weight loss. Many dieters are lacking in CoQ10. In one study, two groups of overweight individuals followed the same *restricted diet*. One group was given a placebo and the other group took 100 mg of CoQ10 a day. Both groups lost weight after 60 days. However, the group taking CoQ10 lost 17 <u>more</u> pounds than the placebo group.

*Milk thistle is an effective liver cleanser and age-proofing antioxidant. It removes toxins from the liver to improve its function and can help regenerate the liver's growth. When the liver functions well, weight loss is easier. Milk thistle contains potent antioxidants silymarin and glutathione to boost the immune system, fight free radicals and prevent oxidative damage. It can provide younger-looking skin and a more rejuvenated body. Some recent research I uncovered revealed that milk thistle may play a part in delaying tumor growth.

*Lecithin can help increase skin elasticity and thickness, improve hair and nail condition and support joint health. Lecithin helps break down cholesterol, helping to lower blood pressure and support heart health. In addition, lecithin can help break down fat in the liver and bloodstream to aid weight loss. Take a lecithin capsule with meals or add 1 tbsp. of organic lecithin powder to a morning protein drink. Enjoy eating chocolate, ladies - it contains lecithin!

*Red rice yeast is a common Chinese cholesterol-lowering and cardio support supplement. Its phytosterols are clinically proven to help support good HDL cholesterol, reduce bad cholesterol and the risk of heart disease. It can also help with weight loss.

*Garlic & cayenne pepper is a powerful antioxidant combination that can help provide better circulation, ignite fat-burning, reduce triglycerides, support healthy cholesterol and can help support heart health. **NOTE:** Do not take garlic supplements if taking blood-thinning medications. Check with your doctor first.

__Probiotics__ support a healthy immune system, encourage better absorption of key minerals and vitamins, aid digestion by helping the body break down fats, protein, carbohydrates and dairy foods, balance friendly bacteria in the intestines, promote regular bowel movement, eliminate harmful bacteria, plaque, bad breath, replenish healthy bacteria (when taking antibiotics), and can help us feel uplifted. Did you know that our intestinal tract contains over 1,200 different types of bacteria that aid digestion? Many doctors feel that taking probiotics may play a role in preventing diseases including Parkinson's, colds and flu, irritable bowel syndrome, diarrhea and more. Taking certain medications, high stress lifestyles, travelling, depression, constipation, and consumption of processed foods can cause ill-health, imbalances in the flora and deplete the intestines of 'good' bacteria. When our flora is balanced, we feel uplifted.

A popular probiotic brand recommended by doctors is **Candidase**, for those with or prone to yeast infections. It contains both cellulose and protease to help break down fungi and prevent overgrowth. Because the inside of the cell of yeast is mostly protein, the protease enzymes *digest* the protein. Cellulase is the only digestive enzyme our body does not make so, when added to our diet, helps the body achieve balance. This brand does not require refrigeration. Keep it in your purse and take two capsules before meals. See more instructions on the bottle. Find it at health foods stores and homeopathic pharmacies.

NOTE: I am often asked for my opinion on supplements and skin care products. At the time of writing this book, I was not paid to endorse the supplements or products I suggest within these pages. See more products noted in **Safe, Effective Face & Body Product Suggestions**.

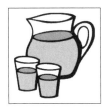

Age-Proofing Tip #52
Importance of Water & Weight Loss

Are you drinking enough water? We've heard it a million times - drink eight glasses of water a day. Once you read the following water facts, you'll want to increase your intake to eight glasses a day! After uncovering the health and weight loss benefits of drinking sufficient water, I set a timer to go off every hour while at work. I religiously drank one eight oz. glass from 9 a.m. to 6 p.m. for three days in a row. The result? I lost three pounds and reduced bloating. Drinking sufficient water has been proven to be one of the easiest and most affordable ways to lose body fat too. Here's why:

*Our kidneys need 64 oz. of water per day in order to function effectively. When the kidneys don't get enough water, then the liver is forced to take over some of the work of the kidneys. However, it's the liver's job to metabolize fat and if aiding the kidneys in doing their job, the liver cannot perform its own job sufficiently - which is metabolizing fat! The result? Weight loss comes to a grinding halt. It's imperative to drink sufficient water, especially when dieting, to eliminate toxins and flush fat and waste. Be sure to drink 64 oz. of water a day.

*If you've lost a lot of weight, but have reached a sudden plateau, your liver may be overloaded with fat. Drinking water helps, but you may need a little extra boost. See my apple cider vinegar and garlic slimming tonic recipe in **Age-Proofing Tip #56 - Boost Your Metabolism.**

*For every 25 pounds of additional weight you are carrying, you'll need to drink additional water. For example if you're 40 to 50 pounds overweight, add two more glasses of water to your daily intake. If you're 75 pounds overweight, add three glasses, and so on.

*Drink additional water when exercising or during hot, summer weather.

*Water hydrates the muscles which gives the skin a more toned look. When losing weight, particularly larger amounts, skin can begin to sag. However, by increasing water intake we can prevent loose-looking skin. When skin cells are hydrated with water, skin looks more youthful and firm.

*Water helps suppress appetite. Drink a glass of water when feeling hungry between meals. Cold water is even better. It enters the system more quickly and burns more calories.

*Water binds to salt. If you consume a lot of salt, and experience water retention, increase your water intake. Are you drinking water but still can't shed pounds? You may be retaining water due to added salt in bottled water. About 95% of the brands I researched on the grocer's shelf contained salt or sodium bicarbonate! Be sure to read all bottled water labels. Another less costly solution than water delivery service or buying bottled water is purchasing your own water ionizer. Just attach it to any regular faucet. A water ionizer transforms regular tap water into ionized alkaline water. It tastes better than most bottled waters. In addition, a water ionizer removes lead, chlorine and other chemicals from tap water, but the minerals remain. Drinking ionized water:

-hydrates the body up to six times more than regular water;
-provides oxygen to the body for more energy; and
-helps relieve seasonal allergies.

NOTE: Tumors are known to grow in an acidic environment. Some experts believe that eating an alkaline-rich diet and drinking pH balanced alkaline water may help halt tumor growth. In addition, some individuals report that drinking alkaline water has relieved them of sore joints.

Purchasing a Water Ionizer: Many water ionizing systems cost an arm and a leg (up to $4000). They were simply too costly for my pocket book. However, my hair stylist told me about a manufacturer who makes quality units for $699 to $1000. Purchasing a water ionizer turned out to be the best decision for my family. Here's why. We were spending over $120 a month for regular bottled water. Purchasing the water ionizer for $1000 lowered our water cost to only $83 a month for one year. After that, the unit was paid for and for the past five years we've enjoyed delicious-tasting, ionized water. I bought mine at HydraHappy.com. FYI, it also makes <u>acid</u> water which is the perfect pH for use on the outside of the body. It works wonders on skin and hair, and makes for an excellent hair rinse. Acid water helps kill bacteria so it's great for those with acne and problem skin. You can water plants with acid water too.

Make your Own Spa Water Beverages

Below are four excellent, thirst-quenching spa beverages that you can make at home.

180

Caffeine and Sugar-Free Lemon Iced Tea

This lemon tea recipe is healthy and easy to make. **Here's what you do:**

Bring a quart of water to boil. Remove from heat, add 6 Celestial Seasonings® Lemon Zinger herbal tea bags (caffeine-free) and let steep. After 20 minutes, remove the tea bags and pour the tea into a large carafe of cool water. Add a natural zero calorie sweetener such as stevia (or not) to taste.

Caffeine-Free Hibiscus Tea

Hibiscus tea is wonderful hot or iced. **Here's what you do:**

For hot tea, place 1 bag in a cup of boiled water and enjoy a nice pre-bedtime beverage. To make iced tea, steep 3 hibiscus tea bags in a cup of boiled water and steep to room temperature. Afterward, transfer the tea and bags to a large carafe, add water and refrigerate. No need to sweeten this tea. It tastes great on its own. Even my husband loves it! Hibiscus is an excellent calming tea and helps cool off the body even during the warmest temperatures.

Time-Saver Citrus Beverage

I'm not a big fan of plain water so this time-saving beverage works well for me. **Here's what you do:**

Fill a large carafe with water. Slice 1 lemon in half. Squeeze the juice of ½ the lemon into the carafe. Then make slices of lemon with the other half and add to the carafe. Let cool and enjoy this refreshing, zero calorie, healthy beverage.

Blueberry Water

My husband and I love blueberry water. We like Trader Joe's® Blueberry Estate. It is a certified organic 100% combination of natural juices including blueberry, white grape juice, apple juice, etc. **Here's what you do:**

Pour one inch of juice in a large glass carafe and fill the remainder of the carafe with water. Refrigerate the juice. Enjoy this tasty, super low-calorie beverage.

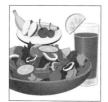

Age-Proofing Tip #53
Super Foods

"Let food be your medicine and medicine be your food." – Hippocrates, Ancient Greek Physician

When we nourish our bodies with healthy foods and exercise, and quiet the mind with prayer and meditation, we become focused and renewed. Eating a variety of colorful fruits and vegetables, hormone-free protein, and healthy fats are essential to peak health and rejuvenation. The foods noted in this section can help curb cravings for sugar or unhealthy carbohydrates, prevent blood sugar spikes, enhance weight loss goals, lower cholesterol, improve the condition of our skin, hair, nails, and provide a feeling of well-being. Add just 30 minutes of daily walking, some stretching and weight resistance exercise and you may shed 10 or more pounds in six weeks!

Whether you're dealing with hormonal imbalances, weight issues, diabetes, or simply want to look and feel younger, the list of super foods noted below can help. **TIP:** Be sure to drink 8-10 glasses of water a day to help flush high fiber foods.

For a more youthful physique, **apples** have been found to contain ursolic acid which builds muscle. Also, according to researchers at *Ohio State University*, apples can reduce bad LDL cholesterol levels by 40%. LDL cholesterol causes tissue damage and inflammation that can lead to plaque buildup and heart attacks. Eating an apple a day (including the peel) <u>can</u> keep the doctor away! Apples are even more effective at lowering bad cholesterol than green tea. However, not all apples are the same. Be sure to choose <u>organic</u> apples as many others are sprayed with toxic pesticides. See my apple mask in **My Favorite Beauty Recipes.**

Powerful, antioxidant-rich **pomegranate** fruit is low in calories and high in vitamin C, fiber, potassium, antioxidants and anti-inflammatory properties than can help defy age, reduce joint inflammation, and fight free radicals. Pomegranate juice halts the formation of plaque in the arteries and breaks down cholesterol. Vitamin C in pomegranates stimulates collagen formation and strengthens blood vessels. One report noted that pomegranates can inhibit the growth of unhealthy cells.

Tasty, low-calorie **blueberries** contain powerful flavonoids (antioxidants) that prevent oxidation and inflammation associated with aging, some cancers and even dementia. They are a low glycemic fruit which is why they're an excellent choice for those watching their weight or challenged with diabetes. The dark color of blueberries is rich in brain-protecting properties that fight free radicals, improve memory and may even prevent the onset of dementia. Blueberries are rich in fiber, vitamin A, and powerful flavonoids that offer four times the antioxidant protection of vitamin C, and 10 times of beta-carotene to boost cardiovascular health. Add blueberries to yogurt, steel cut oats, salad, cereal or a bran muffin recipe. I like to pour frozen blueberries into a morning protein smoothie or my high-protein pancake recipe. See my blueberry protein smoothie, bran muffins and pancake recipe in **My Favorite Healthy Meal & Snack Recipes.**

I am a huge fan of *steel cut oats*. Like my colleague Dr. Alicia Stanton says, "eating oats daily can clean arteries better than some medications." She is the author of, *"The Complete Idiot's Guide to Hormone Weight Loss."* Steel cut oats are the inner portion of the oat kernel. They are minimally processed, have a nuttier taste, and chewier consistency than regular oatmeal. Steel cut oatmeal is a low-glycemic food that enters the blood stream slowly and provides energy, without causing blood sugar spikes. Though it contains starch, the carbohydrates are reduced by the fiber. Steel cut oats offer 10 grams of protein per half-cup serving to help build muscle as well as iron, zinc, and magnesium. In addition, this super food is low in saturated fat and cholesterol, is sodium free, and loaded with soluble fiber that lowers the risk of heart disease. I prefer steel cut oats because they don't cause bloating like regular oatmeal. **NOTE**: Steel cut oats take longer to cook (20-25 minutes for a half cup) than conventional rolled oats.

Yogurt provides millions of beneficial bacteria that can aid digestive issues, boost your immune system, and provide protection against cancer. In addition, it is rich in calcium, protein and vitamin B for bone, muscle and brain support. Choose yogurt brands that offer live and active cultures and avoid those with added fruit as many brands add sugar or high-fructose corn syrup. Try plain greek yogurt which offers much more protein than many other commercial brands. greek yogurt is strained so it offers a thicker, less runny texture. I like to top greek yogurt with chopped apples and walnuts. When in season, I add blueberries, raspberries, or strawberries with 1 tsp. of ground flaxseed, and 1 tsp. raw sunflower seeds, or slivered almonds. Use plain low-fat yogurt to make creamy salad dressings and dips. See my greek yogurt and cilantro dip recipe in **My Favorite Healthy Meal & Snack Recipes**. Non-dairy choices include organic soy, coconut and rice yogurt.

Walnuts are rich in phytonutrients, vitamin E, protein, zinc, magnesium, and are richer in heart-healthy omega 3s than salmon. They offer anti-inflammatory properties such as polyphenols which can lower LDL cholesterol and protect against type II diabetes. Walnuts contain calming properties that make them the perfect snack for those with a busy schedule or high stress occupation. Other nuts offer only one or two of these benefits. A serving of five to eight walnuts is great with apple slices, in salads, sprinkled on yogurt or oatmeal, or with a piece of dark chocolate as a delicious dessert.

Pistachios are one of the lowest calorie nuts. A quarter cup of pistachios (in the shell) is about 90-100 calories. They are rich in protein, fiber, low cholesterol and saturated fats. In addition, pistachios can enhance eye health as they are rich in lutein, caretenoids, calcium, vitamin E, magnesium and zinc.

Almonds are my favorite nut. I eat a handful every day. I keep some in a zip lock bag in my purse, so when going out for a special dinner, I'll eat three to four almonds before biting into a sweet treat. Why? The protein and oils in almonds (all nuts actually) can help prevent blood sugar spikes when eaten prior to a high-glycemic food. Nuts are low in saturated fat and a good source of protein, magnesium, calcium, vitamin A and zinc to improve the look of our skin. Almonds contain plant sterols that reduce absorption of cholesterol too. Other healthy nuts include macadamia (highest in calories), pecans and brazil nuts.

Flax is rich in heart-healthy omega 3 fatty acids and provides a rich source of protein, fiber, zinc and myriad B vitamins. The essential oils in flax can help balance hormones, support the nervous system and stimulate fat burning. Many bodybuilders incorporate flaxseed oil and flax butter into their diets to help build healthy cells and maintain cholesterol levels. Because flaxseeds can help reduce inflammation, they benefit those challenged with sore joints, lupus and other autoimmune diseases. Flaxseed oil is age-defying. Take flaxseed supplements three times a day with meals. Sprinkle ground flax on yogurt, cereal or oatmeal. Find ground flax meal, supplements or combination flaxseed and almond butter at health food stores.

Butternut squash is a fruit, not a vegetable. It is high in fiber and low in fat. It's delicious tasting and loaded with nutrients including carotenes, vitamin A, B6, C, K and potassium. Butternut squash is easy to prepare. See my butternut squash recipe in **My Favorite Healthy Meal & Snack Recipes** and my butternut facial mask in **More Beauty Recipes**.

Broccoli can lower cholesterol and protect eyes from UV rays. It is rich in fiber, carotenoids, vitamin C, K, and folate. In addition, it contains SGS (sulforaphane glucosinolate), a property that is known to prevent cancer growth.

What many don't know is that ***asparagus*** offers even more nutrients than broccoli. It's a superior green vegetable that is rich in vitamin A, K, folate, myriad B vitamins, protein, calcium, fiber, zinc, potassium, selenium and anti-inflammatory agents called saponins that help balance blood sugar levels and provide colon and digestive tract health.

Kale is one of my favorite super foods. It's loaded with health protecting properties that prevent oxidation. Kale is age-defying. It's rich in antioxidants to help fight free radicals, boost our health and reduce cancer risk. It offers anti-inflammatory omega 3 fatty acids, antioxidants A, B, C, E, K, dozens of flavonoids, mood uplifting tryptophan, fiber, calcium, copper, magnesium, manganese, potassium, iron and lutein. Kale triggers the formation of special proteins that keep the arteries free of plaque. Add chopped, raw kale to smoothies and salads, cook it on the stove, or make kale chips. See the delicious kale chip recipe in **My Favorite Healthy Meal & Snack Recipes.**

Spinach is a low-calorie, leafy green that is rich in nutrients including vitamin A, K, iron, folate, manganese, lutein, and plant-based omega 3s. These nutrients can enhance vision, reduce the risk of heart disease, stroke, and osteoporosis. In addition, the folic acid in spinach increases blood flow which provides brain-boosting support. It's low in calories and can be eaten raw in a salad or cooked. Add either cooked or raw spinach to a tomato and cheese omelet for breakfast or add some frozen spinach to a protein and fruit smoothie. Delicious! Try the tasty bean and spinach stew recipe in **My Favorite Healthy Meal & Snack Recipes**.

Romaine lettuce and ***arugula*** are powerful leafy greens that are jam-packed with fiber, vitamins A, C, and K, potassium, folate, iron, magnesium, lutein and calcium. Enjoy a salad once or twice a day topped with healthy dressing such as my favorite garlic/olive oil (GOOD) dressing. Get this healthy, super delicious salad dressing recipe in **My Favorite Healthy Meal & Snack Recipes.**

Avocados are rich in omega 3 fatty acids and antioxidant vitamins B, C and E that can help reduce inflammation such as osteo and rheumatoid arthritis. In addition, avocados contain lutein, lycopene, folate, potassium and magnesium for improved eye health and wellbeing. The healthy fats in avocados are rich in vitamin E and whether eaten or applied topically on skin, avocados can help defy age. Substitute avocado for mayonnaise or serve two slices with eggs for breakfast. Delicious!

Artichokes contain a key ingredient, cynarin, which triggers the stimulation of bile and digestive juices produced by the liver. Bile is a key digestive component that reduces gas, constipation and helps induce regular elimination. As far back as ancient Roman times, artichokes have been used as a digestive aid. Whenever I eat artichokes my skin glows - likely because they also help detoxify the liver.

Sweet potatoes are considered the ultimate nutritional food. They're not only tasty and satisfying; they're rich in fiber, vitamin C, carotenoids and potassium. Just bake and serve one as a satisfying side dish with meats, poultry or egg dishes.

Pumpkin seeds, also known as pepitas, are rich in phytosterols which reduce cholesterol, tryptophan which uplifts the mood, carotenoid antioxidants, minerals including iron, zinc, copper, magnesium and phosphorous, protein and healthy monosaturated fat. Pumpkin seeds offer anti-inflammatory benefits to those challenged with sore joints or arthritis.

Chia seeds are very versatile, nutritional and high in fiber. Just one tbsp. of chia seeds contains 3 grams of protein, omega 3 fatty acids, 6 grams of fiber and only 70 calories. Add them to protein shakes or sprinkle on oatmeal, or a fruit and yogurt bowl. See my recipe for chia pudding and my fantastic low-carb, wheat-free pancake recipe with chia seeds in **My Favorite Healthy Meal & Snack Recipes**.

Black beans protect against free radicals due to their key property, anthocyanin. They are low in calories, high in fiber, protein, iron, biotin, folate and zinc. They are free of saturated fat and can boost brain power, support the heart and reduce inflammation. Black beans are age-defying. Just one half cup provides 8 grams of protein, and 7 grams of fiber. Enjoy black beans as a side dish with eggs, in a breakfast burrito, veggie chili, or salads. Find organic canned black beans in all health food stores and Trader Joe's to name a few.

Lentils are high in nutrients including lean protein, fiber, iron, copper, potassium, folate, magnesium, potassium, vitamin B, and mood-uplifting tryptophan. Lentils help lower cholesterol and triglycerides, prevent blood sugar spikes, constipation, and are fat free.

Garbanzo beans (AKA chickpeas) are high in fiber, protein, antioxidants C and E, beta-carotene, phytonutrients, and minerals such as iron, copper and manganese. Garbanzo beans provide digestive and colon health, balance blood sugar levels and support the heart by lowering cholesterol and triglycerides. They offer mood-calming tryptophan too. Add garbanzo beans to salads, soup, curry, stew, or quinoa. One of my favorite dips, hummus, is made with garbanzo beans. See the tasty hummus recipe in **My Favorite Healthy Meal & Snack Recipes**.

Carrots are low in calories and loaded with nutrients including iron, copper, carotene and vitamins C, E, D and K. They are age-proofing and can help reduce inflammation associated with lupus and rheumatoid arthritis. Substitute carrots for corn chips and dip them into hummus and low-fat yogurt dip. If you have a juicer, add a carrot, an apple, some kale, and celery sticks to make a healthy antioxidant-rich fruit and veggie drink. I place big chunks of carrots around a roast chicken or dice a carrot into little chunks and add them to stew, chili, or soup.

Gluten-free *quinoa* is rich in amino acids and contains more protein than all other grains and vegetables. It offers twice as much protein as brown rice, is rich in anti-inflammatory phytonutrients, vitamin E, quercetin, omega 3 fatty acids, alpha-linolenic acid, and minerals including magnesium, phosphorus, fiber, copper, and folate, to name a few. In addition, it's a tasty comfort food grain that contains mood uplifting tryptophan and age-defying properties that prevent oxidation and inflammation. I consider it the ultimate low-carb grain and it's gluten-free too. I rarely eat rice since discovering the health benefits of quinoa. Find white, red or tri-colored organic quinoa at most health food stores. All three types offer a delightful, nutty taste. It cooks quickly - just 10 minutes. Boil quinoa in water or organic chicken broth. Add your choice of chopped green onions, sliced black olives and feta cheese, or diced sun dried tomatoes, olive oil, walnuts and a sprinkle of parmesan cheese. **NOTE**: Red quinoa is richer in fiber and protein than white.

Nutritional yeast (vegetarian grown) is derived from molasses. It is high in protein, folic acid, B5 (pantothenic acid), B12, B6, zinc, over 15 amino acids, and is low in fat and sodium. I like **KAL Nutritional Yeast Flakes** because they are non-GMO, gluten-free, unsweetened and offer a nutty taste. Add nutritional yeast to soups, smoothies, or dehydrated kale chips. See the recipe for kale chips in **My Favorite Healthy Meal and Snack Recipes**.

Shiritaki noodles are made with dried flour derived from the Asian konjac plant. Shirataki noodles are a healthy, low-calorie, low-glycemic, high-fiber alternative to regular wheat or rice noodles. In addition, they are free of fat, sugar, and gluten. Because they contain soluble fiber and only trace carbohydrates, these noodles are a healthy and satisfying choice for those on low-carb diets or challenged with diabetes. Boiling the noodles softens the texture and activates the fiber (glucomannan) creating a feeling of fullness. In addition, these fiber-rich noodles reduce blood-sugar spikes and can help address constipation. Find both plain shirataki and tofu shirataki noodles in the refrigeration section at most grocery stores. They are packed in water and have a fishy odor. However, rinsing the noodles prior to preparation eliminates the odd smell. Use them in a stir-fry, in soups or with sauces. See the recipe for healthy, carbohydrate-free and delicious ramen-like soup made with these versatile noodles in **My Favorite Healthy Meal and Snack Recipes**.

Sea kelp noodles and roasted seaweed flakes are two staples for those on raw food diets. They are low calorie sources for those with iodine deficiencies. **Sea kelp noodles** are salt-free and contain iodine to help regulate the thyroid hormone and metabolic rate. Sea kelp noodles are very crunchy, so they're best when added to coleslaw and salads. **Roasted seaweed flakes** are crispy 2 x 3 inch seaweed sheets that are roasted with olive or sesame oil and sea salt. They're a delicious iodine-rich snack. Find both products in health food stores. **NOTE:** *Women's Health* reports that 9 out of 10 women who struggle with weight loss, test positive for iodine deficiency. Iodine is vital for thyroid balance. When iodine is adjusted, women lose stubborn pounds and keep the weight off.

Wild salmon is rich in protein and omega 3 fatty acids that help support cardiovascular health and provide age-defying properties for healthy, more youthful-looking skin. The bright orange antioxidant, astaxanthin, helps support joints and relieves inflammation. The natural oils in salmon can enhance memory and brain function. Be sure to avoid farmed salmon as it contains higher levels of PCB contaminants. Choose wild salmon or other low-level contaminated fish such as tuna and mackerel.

Sardines are rich in CoQ10, protein, calcium, potassium, iron, B12, selenium, vitamin D and omega 3 fatty acids. The myriad benefits of sardines include cardiovascular support, improved memory and energy. They also contain tryptophan for mood support. See my sardine and goat cheese snack made with Ryvita®

crispbread rye crackers in **My Favorite Healthy Meal & Snack Recipes.**

Olive oil is rich in anti-inflammatory polyphenols, mono-saturated oleic acid, phytonutrients, vitamin E, and omega 3 and 9 fatty acids. Olive oil supports heart health and can lower blood pressure, risk of diabetes and other diseases. Over two dozen studies conclude that olive oil can reduce the development of many cancers including digestive and respiratory tract, breast and colon. Olive oil reduces oxidation so it's considered one of the healthiest oils. In a French study conducted with a group of senior citizens, those who used olive oil in dressings and for cooking, were found to maintain better memory and concentration than those who used little or no olive oil at all. Whether consumed or applied topically, olive oil is wonderful for our skin. As noted earlier, squalane derived from olives is an effective topical oil for all skin types. It does not clog pores.

Garlic offers myriad health benefits. It is known to help prevent plaque buildup and is a proven cholesterol reducer and fat blocker, according to one study conducted in Israel. Other studies including one from *Arizona State University*, as well as a team of *ASU* scientists agree that garlic can help with weight loss. Remarkably, garlic breaks down fat in the bloodstream before it can enter the cells, which slows the storage of body fat. Garlic supports the digestive system and can help eliminate harmful toxic microbes, hundreds of types of parasites, and yeast that end up in the intestines and gut due to consuming sugar, simple carbohydrates, or contaminated foods. Garlic contains allicin, the powerful property that attacks harmful invaders and is thought to be an excellent yeast infection preventative. Another study in *Healthy Living* noted that garlic can boost immunity. It attacks viruses, bacteria and tumor cells and prevents inflammation which is known to cause aging, heart disease, Alzheimer's and even cancer. Garlic protects the brain and can reduce dementia. It even uplifts us. In addition, garlic contains cancer-killing properties and attacks free radicals used in radiation treatments. Read more about the weight loss benefits of garlic in my slimming tonic recipe noted in **Age-Proofing Tip #56 - Boost Your Metabolism.**

Honey has been linked to longer living and sharper thinking. It contains properties such as quercetin and caffeic acid that improve brain function. Honey contains folate, iron, B vitamins and is known to help lower both triglycerides and cholesterol. Residents of one Greek island, consume honey rather than sugar or artificial sweeteners, and maintain a Mediterranean diet consisting of olives and oil, fresh fish, vegetables and low-glycemic fruits. According to *Nutrient Insider* and the *Journal of Medicinal Food,* by consuming honey that is indigenous to their island, senior citizens experience lower rates of cancer, dementia, heart disease, and enjoy sex in their 80s. Honey offers even more benefits. Consuming locally grown honey is known to help relieve allergies, and when applied topically, it can help heal minor wounds. Honey is a natural antibiotic. Add it to hot tea to prevent a cold and flu. It is an excellent ingredient when used in facial masks. It is a natural hydrator. **NOTE:** Honey is not recommended for children under the age of three.

Chocolate is loaded with skin rejuvenating polyphenols that increase blood flow to the skin. Chocolate contains powerful antioxidant-rich catechins and flavonoids that can reduce the development of some cancers and protect against cardiovascular disease. Flavonoids are the key antioxidants of chocolate because they prevent clots and inflammation. A recent study noted that flavonoids in both milk and dark chocolate can lower bad cholesterol levels and reduce high blood pressure. In addition, chocolate contains mood-lifting properties and lecithin which helps breaks down fat. Enjoy eating chocolate without the guilt.

For more information and up-to-date nutrition and food safety updates visit world's healthiest foods at whfoods.org.

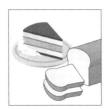

Age-Proofing Tip #54
How the Glycemic Index of Foods
Affect Health & Weight

High Glycemic (GI) Foods

The glycemic index (GI) measures how fast the carbohydrates in a food absorbs into the bloodstream. The higher the number, the greater it increases blood sugar levels, also known as blood sugar spikes. To prevent weight gain, uplift our mood and keep hormones balanced, avoid or reduce consumption of high glycemic index (HGI) foods (AKA high-carbohydrate foods).

Here's why: High-carbohydrate foods enter the system quickly which causes a temporary *high* such as uplifted mood and increased energy. But after an hour or so, the blood sugar takes a drastic dive causing a *crash* effect - resulting in loss of energy, irritability or depression and triggers cravings for <u>more</u> high carbohydrate foods! This vicious cycle messes with our wellbeing and our waistlines! In addition, high GI foods cause water retention, inflammation and aging, diabetes, fibromyalgia pain and increased blood pressure. Avoid or limit high GI foods.

A food with a GI of 70 or more is considered <u>high</u>.

Examples of high glycemic (HGI) foods are white bread and wheat products including many breakfast cereals and bars, bagels, muffins, jams, candy, cakes, ice cream, cookies, white pasta, noodles, white potatoes, brown and white rice, crackers, corn chips, beets, sodas, fruit juices, and alcohol, to name a few. Be sure to read labels on all condiments, sauces, and dips for hidden HGI ingredients such as sugar, potato starch, tapioca, corn and flour.

NOTE: HGI potatoes can cause inflammation associated with sore joints. Unfortunately, many medications and supplements are formulated with potato starch as a binder ingredient. Check medication labels for a list of ingredients.

Low (LGI) and Medium (MGI) Glycemic Foods

Consuming LGI to MGI foods <u>are the best choices for all women</u>, in particular those challenged with brain fog or poor memory, weight gain, water retention, hormonal changes, fatigue, irritability, loss of energy or muscle tone, sadness or depression, diabetes, fibromyalgia, or high blood pressure. LGI and MGI foods release more slowly into the system, preventing blood sugar spikes, and provide a feeling of fullness that lasts for a longer period of time. These foods also reduce cravings for HGI (high carb) foods. By consuming LGI and MGI foods we can improve our health, mood, concentration and energy, balance hormones, prevent fibromyalgia pain, lower blood pressure, speed weight loss goals and reverse diabetes.

A food with a GI of 56 to 69 is considered <u>medium</u> and a GI of 55 or less is <u>low</u>.

Examples of medium glycemic (MGI) foods are butternut and acorn squash, sweet potatoes, radishes, apples, oranges, nectarines, tangerines, cantaloupes, mangos, pears, plums, pineapples and kiwis.

Examples of low glycemic (LGI) foods are cheeses, meat, fish (anchovies, tuna, cod, mackerel, salmon, trout, sole, sardines) shrimp, lobster, scallops, chicken, duck, turkey, venison, lamb, high fiber foods such as lentil, pinto, fava, black, white and green beans, chickpeas, barley, steel cut oats, quinoa, basmati rice, split peas, green peas, lentil flour, almond meal, soy flour, blueberries, blackberries, strawberries, raspberries, grapefruits, and non-starchy vegetables such as romaine and dark leafed lettuces, radicchio, arugula, broccoli, brussel sprouts, artichokes, asparagus, cucumbers, radishes, kale, okra, swiss chard, spinach, mushrooms, onions, chives, parsley, bell peppers, green and red cabbage, celery, avocados, non-GMO (genetically modified organisms) vegetable oils, spices and herbs, avocados, seeds, nuts (walnuts, pistachios, almonds, macadamia nuts), nut butters (flax, cashew, almond) and natural sweeteners such as xylitol, agave and stevia.

Tip: Though we can all benefit from eating low GI carbs at each meal, we <u>can</u> still indulge in a baked treat from time to time. **Here's what you do:**

Combine a high GI baked food with a protein food or low GI nuts and you will lower the overall GI value down to medium. Woo hoo! - Have your cake and eat it too!

For more GI foods and information visit glycemicindex.com

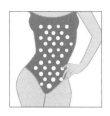

Age-Proofing Tip #55
Slimming Tips

Due to aging, stress, pain, fluctuating hormones, and weight gain, our dietary needs will require some healthy changes by age 40. Some of us tend to overeat or choose foods that offer little nutritional value, especially when feeling stressed or 'blue.' Eating processed, high-carbohydrate foods and trans fats can cause wrinkles and rapid aging, pain, disease, inflammation, irritability, brain fog and added pounds and inches.

To maintain or lose weight, and improve how we look and feel, a few *eating adjustments* can trigger joy, better mental focus, a more toned physique, younger-looking skin, increased energy, and better health and sleep. Regular walking, stretching and weight resistance exercise should also be incorporated. I've noted some revolutionary and practical suggestions in **Age-Proofing Tip #57 - Weight Resistance Exercise** - even if you can't get to the gym. In addition, incorporating high-fiber foods and beneficial supplements can speed results. Below are several healthy tips that can help you eat your way thin and slow down aging.

NOTE: Before making dietary changes or trying the supplements and suggestions noted below, consult with your doctor or a nutritionist if you have concerns or are taking special medications.

*Eat regularly. Schedule your meals and snacks. Choose to eat either three meals and two healthy snacks, or six small meals a day.

*Consume a low-carbohydrate, low-glycemic, high-fiber diet. Many studies have proven that by avoiding wheat, sugar and other starchy, high-carbohydrate foods, we can slow aging, improve memory, prevent brain fog, prevent and reduce pain, disease, and drop pounds far more successfully! Diets such as *The Zone, The Mediterranean Diet* and *Dr. Adkins* basically follow this concept. However, I recommend adding fiber and substituting some foods noted, such as bacon or pork rinds, with less fatty and more nutritional options such as avocados, olives, nuts or organic cottage cheese.

*Do not skip meals. When we do, the body goes into survival mode and slows down metabolizing fat. Consuming few calories during the day leaves us feeling ravenous by evening. This sets us up to 'binge eat' which leads to choosing the wrong foods, and consuming more calories than we need. I strongly suggest removing processed, sugary, starchy, high-carbohydrate foods from your cupboards to avoid temptation.

*Do not watch TV, work on a computer, talk on the phone, read or text while eating meals. These distractions cause mindless eating and gulping. Eating a meal is your time to relax, de-stress and nourish your body.

*Don't eat when in a hurry. Digestion begins in the mouth where saliva enzymes help 'pre-digest' and break down food. Chew food well, especially if your goal is to drop pounds. Become aware of each bite of food by chewing at least 15 times. Slower eating triggers a feeling of fullness and prevents over eating. Try putting eating utensils down between bites to ensure that you take sufficient time to chew.

*Avoid fat-free or sugar-free (artificially sweetened) foods. They are often enhanced with sodium and starches. Also, when fat is removed from foods, we feel less satisfied, which leads to over-eating. Many processed diet foods offer little nutritional value. Eat smaller portions of full-fat foods.

*Limit or avoid diet sodas. They are laden with artificial sugar substitutes that can cause cravings for more soda and more food. If watching your weight, diet soda is not your friend. In addition, drinking more than two sodas daily have been linked to other serious health issues. Read more in **Age-Proofing Tip #15 - Avoid Artificial Sweeteners**.

*When you feel full - stop eating. Try flossing and brushing teeth immediately after eating dinner. This can avoid the temptation to snack prior to bed time.

*Before and after lunch and dinner, sip a cup of green tea. Green tea contains polyphenols including epigallocatechin gallate (EGCG) which increase fat burning. Did you know that drinking one cup of green tea *before meals* can help you drop up to 10 pounds over the course of one year? Even better - drinking it *before and after* each meal of the day can reduce weight by up to 15 pounds in a year! If you don't like the taste of green tea, consider taking green tea extract in capsule form. See ***Thermo Green Tea*** capsules in **Safe, Effective Face & Body Product Suggestions.**

*Drink water or tea instead of eating between meals. Quite often we mistake hunger for dehydration and reach for food rather than a nice, tall glass of water. If you're not a fan of water, enhance the flavor with a slice of lemon or sip on caffeine-free herbal teas or organic, low-sodium organic chicken broth.

*Diuretic teas such as dandelion or rosemary can help reduce water retention and can help clear blemishes and acne.

*Send the bread basket back to the kitchen when eating out. Instead of starchy bread, order a small side salad while waiting for your entrée. If planning to eat a starchy meal, the vinegar in salad dressing helps prevent blood sugar spikes. Or drink my slimming tonic prior to each meal of the day. Read more about it in **Age-Proofing Tip #56 - Boost Your Metabolism.**

*If you choose to snack, select medium and low-glycemic fruits and veggies and combine them with nuts or protein to maintain steady blood sugar levels. For example, apple slices dipped in 1 tbsp. almond butter or carrot sticks with hummus. See more snacks in **My Favorite Healthy Meal & Snack Recipes.** Read more about low and medium glycemic index foods in **Age-Proofing Tip #54.**

*Eating high-fiber foods stabilizes blood sugar levels and creates a feeling of fullness. Consuming high-fiber foods also reduces the risk of bowel and colon cancer. Include two cups of vegetables/high-fiber foods with lunch and dinner.

*Weight loss is nearly impossible when constipated. Quite often constipation is the result of not drinking enough water, especially if you've increased your intake of high fiber foods. Fiber + dehydration = bloating that 'stops us up,' hindering weight loss efforts. Increase water intake to 10-12 glasses of water a day to help flush fiber, toxins, and fats from your system. Sufficient water prevents bloating and improves elimination. Take a moment to review **Age-Proofing Tip #48 - Relieve Constipation, Bloating & Gas.**

Fats, Oils & Nuts

*Avoid trans fats (AKA hydrogenated oils). They are artificially hardened to remain solid at room temperature. Hydrogenated fats are added to many commercially-processed foods because they help preserve their shelf life. They are usually noted as hydrogenated palm, cottonseed or corn oil (just to name a few). These fats are not easily digested and hinder our weight loss efforts. They slow down fat burning because they clog our blood, cause oxidation (which ages us), increase bad cholesterol, affect insulin production and cause cardiovascular disease.

*Choose unsaturated oils such as extra virgin cold-pressed organic olive, safflower, sunflower, walnut, grape seed or coconut oil. They are much healthier choices that the body can digest. Make my husband's (GOOD) salad dressing recipe noted in **My Favorite Healthy Meal & Snack Recipes.** It's delicious on salads, steamed veggies, poultry, meats and fish.

*Consume healthy seeds, nuts and oils such as flax, pumpkin, almond, walnut, pistachio and brazil nuts. Almond butter or flaxseed/almond butter are excellent choices too. However, choose nuts that are packed in sealed bags. Do not purchase nuts (or grains) that are sold in open bins as they are found to be either contaminated with germs or may contain mold that is carcinogenic. One cardiologist I interviewed highly recommends one to two brazil nuts a day. They are rich in selenium, help uplift mood and reduce plaque in the arteries.

Protein and Processed Meats

*Eat 6 oz. of protein with three meals a day. Protein helps maintain lean muscle mass. It's the primary building block of muscle which helps keep our bodies looking toned and more youthful. In addition, the more muscle we have, the more rapidly we can burn calories. Choose low-fat proteins and dairy products that are free of antibiotics and hormones. Grass fed beef is lower in saturated fat, therefore considered one of the best red meats. Six ounces of meat is about the size of the palm of your hand and ¾ to 1" thick. Other sources of protein include eggs, soy, cheese, tofu, poultry, fish, beans, nuts and nut butters.

*Cut back on processed, fatty meats such as bacon, pastrami, ribs, etc. to reduce abdominal fat, high cholesterol, and high blood pressure. Hormones in these foods may be associated with weight gain and hormone imbalance.

Avoid Wheat

Bread is a naturally high glycemic food. Eating bread frequently can cause myriad health issues from weight gain to unbalanced hormones, fatigue, fibromyalgia, moodiness, depression, diabetes, inflammation, pain, aging and cravings for more carbs. Many physicians and health experts believe that eliminating wheat altogether may be valid. One reason is that wheat causes cravings for more carbohydrates. In addition, over 80% of women cannot properly digest gluten, a common ingredient found in wheat. It causes bloating, yeast problems, water retention, weight gain and difficulty losing weight. A recent report in *Nutrient Insider* noted that gluten can contribute to high blood pressure.

For this reason, many women have switched to gluten-free bread. However, <u>gluten-free breads also cause weight gain</u> because they are made with high GI (Glycemic Index) starchy flours such as potato, rice, and corn which cause blood sugar spikes. So, gluten-free breads are not the answer for those with weight issues. To avoid weight gain and health issues, switch to non-starchy flours such as almond and hazelnut meal or garbanzo and coconut flour. Find Bob's Red Mill® almond, hazelnut, coconut and garbanzo flours at many health food stores.

If you love pasta and rice, stock up on shirataki noodles. I also like tofu shirataki angel hair noodles. Shirataki noodles are delicious. They contain only 20 calories a serving, are free of gluten, sugar, and wheat, and are high in fiber. The trace carbohydrates in these versatile noodles are so low, that when you subtract the fiber and protein from the total carbs, the net carbs equal zero. Use both noodles in place of pasta or in soups and stir fries. Read more about these healthy noodles in **Age-Proofing Tip #53 - Super Foods** and check out the wheat-free 'ramen' noodle recipe in **My Favorite Healthy Meal & Snack Recipes.** Another good rice substitute is high protein, gluten-free organic quinoa.

Baking Tip: If you like baking, try reducing the carbohydrate level of your baked treat by reducing the flour portion of the recipe. To do this, substitute wheat flour with almond or hazelnut meal (100% ground nuts), soy bean, coconut or garbanzo bean flours. Nut meal flours taste delicious and add moisture and good fat to baked goods. In addition, you will prevent blood sugar spikes and weight gain. Those who use gluten-free flour may consider substituting half or more for nut flour when baking. Nut flours drop the carbohydrate and glycemic index to much healthier levels. See my delicious high-fiber, low-carb and low-glycemic blueberry bran muffin recipe in **My Favorite Healthy Meal & Snack Recipes.** It's THE best bran muffin ever! Be sure to also try my flour-free protein pancake recipe. It's delicious!

*Snacking on a **natural, high-protein bar** can come in handy. However, many so-called healthy protein bars contain sugar, artificial sweeteners, gluten, corn syrup and other not-so-healthy ingredients. For years I've been on the search for a protein bar that is naturally sweetened. And I finally found one! It's the **Quest®** bar, made with 100% natural ingredients, 20 grams of protein, high fiber, contains no sugar, artificial sweeteners or sugar alcohols, is gluten-free and sweetened with lo han guo and stevia! It's delicious. I love the lemon cream pie and coconut cashew. Get them at select health food stores.

*Are you taking medication for heart disease and/or high blood pressure? Several of these medications can actually raise insulin levels! When insulin levels are high, the body stores fat, resulting in weight gain and higher blood pressure! It's a catch-22! Consistently high insulin levels can also eventually lead to diabetes! The good news is high blood pressure can be reduced by incorporating a low carbohydrate diet as noted earlier in this section. A low-carbohydrate diet helps the body attack stored fat and lowers blood pressure. I think it best to avoid eating wheat if challenged with high blood pressure. Discuss the suggestions noted in this book with your doctor. Also, be sure to mention the supplements noted, as well as my slimming tonic in **Age-Proofing Tip #56 - Boost Your Metabolism**. It helps clear a fatty liver. **NOTE:** Many doctors prescribe meds because it's easier and faster than sitting down and writing out a diet plan for each patient. The bottom line is... you are responsible for your own health and happiness. It takes persistence and dedication, but I guarantee that by adjusting your eating habits you will improve your health and look and feel younger. Consider switching doctors or see a nutritionist if your healthcare professional insists on prescribing drugs for blood pressure issues.

The following books explain in more detail how to maintain blood pressure without drugs, reduce weight and rejuvenate the skin by incorporating a low-carbohydrate diet. *The Zone*, *South Beach Diet* and the *Mediterranean Diet* are all worth reading because they are all based on low-carb eating. Find these books at your local library or bookstore.

*Read about vitamin D and resveratrol - two timely, scientifically proven supplements that can help with rapid weight loss, protect health, uplift mood, protect against certain cancers, and much more in **Age-Proofing Tip #51 - My Favorite Supplements for Women.**

*Omega 3 flaxseed and plant-based omega 6s can help lower blood sugar levels, ignite fat burning, uplift our mood and enhance overall wellbeing. Read more details about plant-based omega 3s and omega 6s in **Age-Proofing Tip #51 - My Favorite Supplements for Women.**

*Many adults cannot digest lactose found in milk and dairy products, causing bloating and weight gain. Look for lactose-free products or consider taking a lactase supplement to help break down milk sugar. Essential digestive enzymes, taken before or with foods, can help break down protein, fats, carbohydrates, as well as milk sugar. Find them at your local health food store. Milk substitutes are rice, soy or almond milk.

*Do not eat fats or carbs before bed. If feeling hungry at bedtime, make a protein drink with a scoop of whey protein, ice and water. Be sure the protein mix does not contain sugar.

*According to a study performed by the *National Institute of Health*, chewing gum between meals can help keep weight off. It stimulates your 'feel full' hormones which helps reduce grazing between meals. See healthy gum suggestions in **Age-Proofing Tip #39 - Brighter Pearly Whites. NOTE:** Chewing gum is known to cause bloating and gas.

Holiday Season Slimming Tip

Holiday time means that chocolates, cookies and alcoholic beverages are everywhere in sight. Enjoying a sweet treat or drink from time to time is okay. When you want to indulge in a decadent dessert or cocktail, you can prevent extra holiday pounds by incorporating the following suggestions.

1. The order in which you eat certain foods can prevent blood sugar spikes and weight gain. **Here's what you do:**

Before consuming a high carbohydrate food or drink, eat a little bite of protein or fat first. For example; four or five almonds or a slice of cheese. By consuming the protein/fat in the nuts or cheese first, the high carbohydrates consumed afterwards will enter the bloodstream more slowly, preventing blood sugar spikes and weight gain.

2. Read about my popular apple cider vinegar and garlic slimming tonic in **Age-Proofing Tip #56 - Boost Your Metabolism.** In a nutshell, drinking the slimming tonic prior to meals prevents the fat in the blood stream from entering the fat cells. The tonic also reduces food cravings, bloating, food poisoning, and more. The weight loss and health benefits of this *pre-meal* dynamic duo are incredible. I've noted a life-changing story below of how one woman lost over 200 lbs. with the help of the slimming tonic.

An Inspiring Story – How One Woman Dropped Over 200 Pounds!

This is an inspiring story you're sure to enjoy. In April 2011, I was a guest speaker at The Women's Expo in Nevada. While there, an energetic woman came running up to me waving a photo in one hand and a copy of my book, *"Hollywood Beauty Secrets: Remedies to the Rescue,"* in the other. She said, "I had to meet you in person because you helped change my life!"

She introduced herself as Coralynn and she revealed a photo of herself at 400 lbs.! She said, "At this weight, I was taking OVER 17 medications for diabetes, blood pressure, cholesterol, heart and other health issues. And I dragged an oxygen tank with me 24/7. People stared, pointed, made jokes, and called me names. I've been teased almost all of my life. No one knows how tough it was on me - but I just kept smiling. Luckily my husband has always loved me regardless of my weight. But the turning point for my weight loss was the day he told me that we would no longer be taking vacations. With my difficulty walking, he would have to haul the oxygen tanks and medications. And now he no longer wanted to take road trips and cruises. Our trips were no longer a vacation for him. But I lived to travel - that was my passion! And I knew right at that moment I had to make some changes. At 400 lbs. I couldn't even get down on my knees to pray. So I sat in my chair and asked God to help me take charge of my health."

Coralynn then shared her weight loss plan with me. She began by reading books about nutrition, then reduced the size of her food portions, and stuck to a low carbohydrate diet. She took control of her life! Within a year Coralynn had dropped a whopping 100 pounds, getting down to 300 lbs. She was now able to walk a little, but not enough to budge past the plateau weight of 300. Her liver was now full of fat which halted her weight loss.

But keeping her positive spirit, she stayed on track searching for more answers. And one day, Coralynn saw me on a TV show making some natural beauty recipes. She ordered a copy of my book and used many of my tips, and had a discussion with her doctor about my slimming tonic recipe. He agreed that it would help clear the fat from her liver. My doctor-approved slimming tonic, which I had learned from my mother, landed me on the cover of Woman's World Magazine. See the recipe in **Age-Proofing Tip #56 - Boost Your Metabolism.**

So now, here was Coralynn standing in front of me just one year later. She was beaming, full of life, and looked nothing like her photo. With the help of the slimming tonic, and eating healthy foods, Coralynn had dropped another 140 pounds for a total weight loss of 240 lbs.!! And she reduced her medications from 17 down to only ONE! I was on the verge of tears and said, "Coralynn - I am so proud of you! Thank you for sharing your story. YOU did this! You made the choice and took the steps to transform your health and life."

When I gave my speech later that day, I spotted Coralynn in the audience and invited her up to the podium to tell her story. And she ended her story by turning proudly toward me and said, "I did this for ME!" The crowd clapped and whistled after hearing her life-changing decision to love herself and to make time for her needs. There wasn't a dry eye in the place. Her story will no doubt inspire others who struggle with health, weight or self-esteem issues. She is a role-model. Since meeting Coralynn she has dropped even more weight.

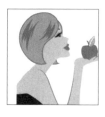

Age-Proofing Tip #56
Boost Your Metabolism

Below are some excellent tips that can help boost your metabolism. **NOTE:** Check with your physician before taking the supplements noted below if you are on medications or have any health concerns.

Apple Cider Vinegar & Garlic Slimming Tonic

A study conducted at *Duke University* notes that, "when too many carbohydrates are consumed, the liver converts them to fat resulting in fatty liver disease." Fatty liver disease hinders weight loss. To help reverse this challenge, incorporate a low-carbohydrate diet and read the benefits of my famous apple cider vinegar (ACV) and garlic slimming tonic. This doctor-approved recipe has helped many individuals eliminate fat in the liver and ignite fat loss.

My parents are living proof that this recipe works. Both Mom and Dad each dropped about 15 to 20 lbs. and they have kept the weight off for over 16 years. Another interesting fact is that they used to suffer from stomach problems, indigestion and ulcers. Since taking this beverage, they no longer have these ailments. They currently take the tonic each morning, prior to breakfast, to maintain their weight loss and health. Read the benefits of both ingredients below.

NOTE: Although my slimming tonic is doctor-recommended, be sure to check with your doctor before taking garlic, especially if currently taking blood-thinning medications.

Health Benefits of Apple Cider Vinegar

Apple cider vinegar (ACV) contains 19 minerals including potassium, phosphorus, magnesium, calcium, sulfur and iron. A pre-meal dose of ACV controls hunger and cravings for sugar, and jumpstarts the metabolism. In addition, ACV prevents blood sugar spikes and contains enzymes that block carbohydrates, preventing starches from entering the system. It can even help prevent food poisoning.

Health Benefits of Garlic

A study conducted in Israel revealed that garlic is a proven cholesterol reducer and fat blocker. **Here's how it works:** Garlic breaks down fat in the blood stream before it can enter the cells, which slows the body's production/storage of fat. Garlic supports the digestive system and can help eliminate harmful toxic microbes, hundreds of types of parasites, and yeast that can make their way into the system via sugar, carbohydrates or contaminated foods and liquids. Garlic can also help prevent a yeast infection due to allicin, a property that protects us from harmful invaders.

An article in *Healthy Living* notes that garlic can reduce plaque buildup and boost immunity. It attacks viruses, bacteria and tumor cells. It prevents inflammation which is known to cause aging, heart disease, Alzheimer's and even cancer. Garlic protects the brain and can reduce dementia. A Russian study noted that garlic offers cancer-killing properties.

In addition, garlic prevents blood sugar spikes and is an energy booster, as proven in a Japanese study. Those administered garlic supplements were less fatigued during and after exercise. According to *UCLA researchers*, garlic can cut stomach cancer risk and slows the hardening of arteries which may help prevent strokes and heart disease. Some super models are known to eat garlic to help with weight loss.

I like Kyolic® brand because it's made with an aged, odorless extract that is powerful and less offensive than regular garlic supplements.

NOTE: Before taking garlic, check with your physician if you are taking blood thinners, medications or have health concerns.

Weight Loss & Health Benefits of <u>Combining</u> Apple Cider Vinegar and Garlic

Combining apple cider vinegar and garlic oil capsules prior to meals can:

-prevent fat in the blood stream from entering the fat cells;
-ignite fat-burning by 'cleansing' the liver. When the liver is free of toxins and fat buildup it can burn fat more efficiently;
-regulate water balance and prevent fluid retention and bloating;
-prevent a buildup of plaque and fatty deposits in the arteries;
-promote oxygenation of the blood;
-calm eczema;
-prevent and clear acne and blemish breakouts;
-reduce the look of cellulite;
-promote healthy cell and tissue growth;
-prevent blood sugar spikes;
-prevent food cravings;
-protect against potent bacteria and viruses such as colds and flus;

-help eliminate yeast overgrowth;
-reduce constipation;
-halt a sore throat;
-help thin blood and lower blood pressure;
-promote wound healing;
-help destroy fungi and prevent food poisoning (when taken prior to a meal);
-provide antiseptic and antibiotic effects; and
-offer over 200 disease-fighting compounds relating to herpes I, herpes II, parasites, bacteria, and fungi.

My Slimming Tonic Recipe

This recipe is safe to use on a long-term basis. **Here's what you do:**

Pour 1 tbsp. organic apple cider vinegar into a 10 oz. glass of water and stir. With that, take approximately 400-600 mg capsule of odorless organic garlic oil.

Slimming Tonic User Tips

To help reduce weight and ignite fat burning, drink this combination <u>before each meal</u> (breakfast, lunch and dinner). If the vinegar mixture is too strong, start with 1 tsp. of apple cider vinegar and within one week, work your way up to 1 tbsp. If you can't tolerate the taste, try adding a little stevia or raw honey to the water/ACV and warm slightly in the microwave. Then drink it down with the garlic capsule. If you're not fond of drinking the AC vinegar, you can find apple cider vinegar capsules at your local health food store. I also suggest making salad with AC vinegar, olive oil and crushed garlic, though taking the slimming tonic prior to meals provides faster results.

In addition, when taken one hour after the last meal of the day, the slimming tonic can help reduce acid reflux for better sleep.

NOTE: For those with more than 30 pounds of weight to lose, or if the liver has become congested with fat as a result of recent weight loss, consider taking the tonic before each meal <u>and snack</u> of the day until you reach your weight loss goal.

Green Tea

Several years ago, I read about the weight loss effects of drinking green tea on an empty stomach (first thing in the morning). I drank the green tea each morning and dropped five pounds in about six weeks. Others report losing up to 15 pounds in one year by drinking green tea *before* and *after* three meals a day. In addition, green tea offers skin rejuvenating and health-boosting benefits. It is rich in anti-inflammatory agents that fight free radicals, protect our health, smooth, firm and hydrate skin, provide additional UV protection, boost memory power, lower cholesterol, and fight disease. I urge you to drink green tea if you have a stubborn metabolism, cholesterol issues, wish to feel better, or achieve younger-looking skin.

Though I am not a fan of the taste of green tea, I like **Natural Organic Raw Green Bush Tea by The Republic of Tea**®, sweetened with a little natural stevia. If you're a coffee drinker, try **Fat Burner Blast Off Coffee**. It's 100% organic fair trade dark roasted coffee beans combined with organic green tea. Enjoy your coffee with the extra antioxidants and fat burning effects of green tea.

Another green tea alternative is taking two **Thermo Green Tea**™ capsules before breakfast and lunch. This gentle, fat-oxidizing formula is 100% ephredra-free and will not cause irritability. Read more about green tea in **Age-Proofing Tip #51 - My Favorite Supplements for Women.**

Green Coffee Bean Extract

Popular *green coffee bean* extract is known to help enhance weight loss goals. But it's not the caffeine in the green coffee bean that stimulates weight loss! The key compound is chlorogenic acid, found in the *raw*, unroasted green coffee bean. Roasting destroys chlorogenic acid (CA). Studies reveal that green extract supports healthy blood sugar levels. According to the *American Journal of Clinical Nutrition*, CA reduces the sugar (glucose) absorption of digested foods when they reach the intestines. It inhibits an enzyme in the liver that releases sugar into the bloodstream. Other studies note that CA can reduce the size of fat cells, stimulate thermogenic fat burning and help control appetite. Take coffee bean extract 20-30 minutes prior to breakfast and lunch to inhibit post-meal glucose levels and improve metabolism. Find **Windmill's Green Coffee Bean Extract** caplets with 50% CA in GNC stores. **NOTE:** Check with your physician before taking this extract especially those with endocrine, kidney, liver, prostate or other health issues.

Trans-resveratrol

You've likely heard the buzz about resveratrol found in red grape skins and seeds. However, *trans-resveratrol*, derived from a root called knotweed, contains even MORE powerful phytonutrients. *Harvard researchers* and countless other studies reveal that trans-resveratrol can add years to our lives. Trans-resveratrol contributes to our overall health and wellbeing because it offers powerful anti-inflammatory agents that slow aging, fade age spots, speed weight loss, reduce pain, increase our energy, and help us look and feel younger. Some women report weight loss when they take it with three meals a day. The dosage required for weight loss is 50-500 ml. a day. Trans-resveratrol offers even more benefits. It can:

-lower blood sugar and improve insulin levels;
-metabolize the release of stored fat when combined with anti-oxidants;
-trigger the muscles to burn fat even more efficiently;
-help curb our appetite;
-help lower blood pressure;
-provide anti-inflammatory compounds that are both anti-aging and reduce pain;
-improve joint health and support cartilage;
-enhance heart health and promote blood flow;
-clear arteries and increase blood flow to the brain to enhance the memory;
-reduce cholesterol and promote flexible arteries;
-increase energy and improve our coordination and circulation; and
-enhance vision.

NOTE: Trans-resveratrol has no known side effects - even at higher doses. Avoid brands that note resveratrol 'blend' on the label. Blends are combined with filler ingredients and are not as potent as pure trans-resveratrol.

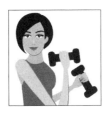

Age-Proofing Tip #57
Weight Resistance Exercise

According to an article noted in *Better Nutrition*, we lose approximately one pound of muscle per year. By age 50, muscle loss rapidly increases which can result in bone fractures and loss of strength.

Exercise is a natural stress buster and mood booster that enhances our health and increases energy. After age 40, weight resistance exercise should be incorporated to help maintain a more youthful looking physique and improve our mental wellbeing. The trick is to lift and lower weights at a super slow rate (5 seconds up and 5 seconds down). This ensures that we use muscle, rather than momentum, to left the weights. Slower weight lifting also prevents stress on joints and torn ligaments.

The *American Diabetes Association* reports that weight resistance exercise just twice a week improves muscle tone and stimulates fat burning. Additional studies have proven that an average woman who strength trains two to three times a week for eight weeks will drop over three pounds of fat and gain two pounds of muscle. Weight resistance exercise can also lower risk of heart disease, increase the endorphins (feel-good transmitters) and improve sleep.

According to *Women's Health Letter*, the average post-menopausal woman loses 3% to 9% of bone mass yearly and over 300,000 women a year experience a hip fracture, due to osteoporosis. Did you know that just 10 minutes of weight resistance exercise each day can prevent and reverse bone loss? You won't need to lift heavy weights or go to the gym! Just 10 minutes of daily *isometric resistance movements* will do the trick. In fact, one study noted that after just two months of isometric exercise, women's bone density rose 7%. See some exercises noted below and be sure to read **Age-Proofing Tip #58 - Body Vibration Plates**, for rapid muscle toning, weight loss, and preventing bone loss.

Exercise Can turn back the Clock

With age, the metabolism becomes sluggish and muscle mass rapidly decreases. By age 40, when our production of human growth hormone (HGH) has drastically declined, we experience signs of aging such as low energy and libido, loose skin, moodiness, anxiety, sleeplessness, gray hair and a sluggish metabolism. Many women and men experience fat deposits on the tummy and others suddenly look or feel older than their years which can sometimes trigger depression or hopelessness.

Exercise improves our confidence, uplifts us, builds stronger muscle, prevents depression, increases bone density, and lowers joint injuries, high blood pressure and risk of heart disease. Let's face it, when we look good, we feel good - and vice versa!

Weight Resistance Stimulates HGH and Builds Bone

Incorporating weight resistance exercise triggers an increase in our <u>natural</u> production of HGH. When HGH is stimulated, muscle tone becomes more defined, the skin looks firmer, libido increases, we sleep better and feel uplifted throughout the day. HGH is responsible for converting amino acids that support the immune system and help build muscle and bone. Muscle stimulates the metabolism so the more muscle we have, the more efficiently we burn fat.

NOTE: Exercise helps the body continue to burn calories for several hours <u>after</u> working out!

In addition to weight resistance exercise, incorporating cardio exercise such as walking 45 minutes, three times a week can ignite fat burning and uplift our mood. Regular exercise decreases stress and halts the production of cortisol (the cause of fat deposits). As noted in **Age-Proofing Tip #16**, getting eight hours of uninterrupted sleep halts cortisol and stimulates more human growth hormone (HGH) production which can enhance our weight loss goals and results in a more youthful-looking appearance.

Be sure to eat protein at each meal to help maintain muscle. Protein includes meat, cheese, nuts and nut butters, beans, eggs, yogurt, tofu, tempeh, venison, lamb, poultry, beans and legumes. Not a meat eater? Choose beans such as garbanzo, black, fava, navy, white, pinto, or lentil, in addition to egg whites, soybeans, tempeh, tofu, yogurt, fish, nuts and nut butters as protein sources.

TV & Exercise

It's a fact that sitting for long periods of time (watching TV or in front of a desk) can cause health issues such as heart disease, bad circulation, weight gain and even depression. Quick bursts of exercise can help prevent and reverse many of these concerns. During a commercial break or once an hour even while at work, incorporate the following exercises. Each one works several muscle groups for speedy results.

Full Body Toner (Stomach, Shoulders, Thighs & Back)

You won't need a pool to perform this fast and easy swimmer's full body toning exercise. All you do is mimic swimming while standing and using your arms! It's one of the easiest ways to quickly achieve toned and defined abs, torso, thighs, shoulders and back. **Here's what you do**:

NOTE: While performing this exercise, <u>engage stomach and thigh muscles</u> to support the back, and sculpt rock hard abs and thigh muscles.

1. Stand with feet hip width apart, arms extended straight out at chest level, and palms facing down with thumbs touching.

2. Bend your knees into a slight squat position while sticking your butt out.

3. While remaining in a squat, circle your right arm DOWN, back and around to the front position, mimicking a swimming stroke. Then alternate with your left arm swinging down, back and around to the front for a total of 30 strokes on each arm.

4. Do a reverse stroke (a back stroke) by circling your right arm UP, back and around in the opposite direction. Alternate with your left arm for a total of 30 strokes on each arm.

Swing a Kettle Ball

Swinging a kettle ball can help tone arms, back, legs, abs and buttocks very quickly. Purchase a 10 lb. kettle ball at any sporting goods store or at a discount department store like TJ Maxx or Marshalls. **Here's what you do:**

NOTE: While performing this exercise keep the stomach muscles engaged.

1. Squat with legs a little wider than hip width apart. Hold the kettle ball between your legs, using both hands.

2. Swing the kettle ball up (with both hands), and come up into a standing position. Squeeze butt and thigh muscles when in the <u>up</u> position.

3. Then, swing the kettle ball back down between the legs and squat down.

4. Repeat 3 sets of 15 reps. This is a very fast and effective exercise.

Butt Lifters

Exercise #1 – Standing Butt Lifter

1. Begin by standing with heels together and toes pointing out, like step one of a ballet plie.

2. Bend the knees, lift heels (keeping heels pressed together) and rise up onto toes. While holding this position, do 12 pelvic tilts. Squeeze the buttocks and stomach muscles each time you tilt the pelvis up.

3. Then, straighten your legs while keeping heels up, and do 15 squats. As you squat up and down, keep abs engaged and squeeze buttock and thigh muscles each time. Do two more sets of 15 for a more firm, raised butt.

Exercise #2 – Horizontal Butt Squeeze (do this exercise at home)

1. Lay on your back with knees bent a little wider than hip width apart and feet flat. Point toes out and place arms by both sides.

2. Keeping feet in place, lift the butt up and squeeze it tightly for 3 seconds when in the up position. Then release. Repeat the up and down movement without touching the butt to the floor. NOTE: Engage abs while doing this exercise. Repeat three sets of 15.

Elliptical Climbers

Elliptical climbers can do wonders for the legs and butt. However, they are quite expensive and rather large for home use. For this reason, I am a fan of the **Air Climber**® which is a heavy duty portable stepper. My sister introduced me to this handy workout device. She says it's one of the speediest ways to firm the butt. I have to agree with her. I can't help 'butt' notice her perky, firm bum when she walks out of a room. Simply stand on the Air Climber® and pump for 50 -100 reps during a commercial break. It's lightweight and easy to store. This weight resistance exercise is sure to get your thighs and butt into peak shape prior to summer. Enjoy wearing shorts ladies!

Pilates

Pilates, developed by Joseph Pilates, is a series of sculpting exercises that define muscles, help flatten the abs, firm and lift buttocks, elongate legs, slim the hips and tone arms. This exercise involves controlled resistance movements that will have your body transformed within weeks. Because of its popularity, Pilates is available in private classes and group sessions in most cities. After taking a few classes you may want to invest in a good quality pilates reformer machine for home use. Aero Pilates® is a nice brand that is priced affordably.

Yoga

Yoga is an excellent form of exercise that is calming, yet effectively strengthens and tones muscles, and increases our energy. It's one of the best forms of exercise for busy women on the go, those experiencing sleeplessness, stress or going through hormonal changes. Yoga involves a series of controlled poses and stretches while focusing on deep breathing, which allows us to get in touch with our spiritual side. Yoga is a gentle, yet powerful, exercise for all women and men. It lowers blood pressure, increases flexibility and is rejuvenating. It can even help reduce cortisol to help support our weight loss goals. Several yoga poses can be performed on a body vibration plate. Read more about them below.

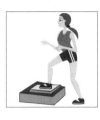

Age-Proofing Tip #58
Body Vibration Plates

With our lives being busier than ever, many of us have limited time and energy to get to the gym. Aging and stress reduces our natural production of HGH resulting in weight gain, sagging skin, and loss of muscle tone especially around the waist, buttocks and thighs. But the great news is that in just 10 minutes a day, you can improve how you look and feel - faster than ever before - with age-defying whole body vibration technology - in the privacy of your own home!

If you're a busy woman or man on the go, a **Body Vibration Plate** machine is the ultimate body transforming solution that quickly sculpts and tones muscles with less stress than lifting weights - in just minutes! In addition, it can help build bone density, balance hormones, boost our mood, smooth cellulite, and more. Read the many health benefits of affordable, muscle-sculpting **Body Vibration Plates** below. I predict that every household will have a vibration plate in coming years. I recently heard that several spas now offer body vibration plate therapy at a cost of $15 to $50 per session.

Not Just for the Elite

A vibration plate is no longer for the elite; it's the affordable answer for stay-at-home moms, baby boomers and busy, working women and men. I was introduced to a Body Vibration Plate back in the mid-90s, when Madonna first had one. However, at that time, it was so costly that only rock stars, professional athletes, super models and movie stars could afford one. Then in 2011, I located a direct distributor of high quality Body Vibration Plates that everyone can now afford. My sisters, friends and countless of my readers have since enjoyed the body-transforming results of this powerful vibration plate.

Compared to traditional training methods such as weight lifting, aerobics or jogging, incorporating vibration plate technology daily achieves better results in far less time with less effort!

Who uses body a vibration plate?

Madonna *Courtney Cox *Elle MacPherson *Mark Wahlberg *Olympic and professional athletes, models, rock stars, NASA astronauts, and me - just to name a few!! It's now affordable so everyone can enjoy the benefits.

How does it work?

The effectiveness of a vibration machine is the superior muscle-activation. A Body Vibration Plate provides smooth, steady oscillation (vibration) which oxygenates the body and triggers a rapid contraction of the muscles between 25 and 50 times per second. The quick contractions stimulate the muscles, accelerating them to burn large amounts of energy and reduce stored fat cells. The rapid vibration stimulates up to 100% of our muscle fibers - unlike normal exercise. Jogging uses only 50%-70% of our muscle fibers. Many doctors agree that the rapid vibration 'shakes' the dormant fat cells to help them release fat. Standing on a vibration plate for just 10-20 minutes allows you to burn far more calories than doing a conventional one hour workout at the gym.

To achieve rapid muscle toning simply squeeze each muscle group (thighs, calves, stomach, butt, arms, etc.) for 60 second intervals. For example, while standing on the plate, hold a static squat and squeeze the thigh muscles for 60 seconds. You may wish to perform a series of squats for 60 seconds or simply hold a lunge while squeezing the legs muscles. Next, stand on toes and squeeze the butt for 60 seconds. Hold a push up, then a crunch - you get the idea. I also recommend sitting on the plate with legs extended and toes pointed. Be sure to engage stomach muscles when performing each position. I've noted a series of positions (a general workout) below. After just minutes a day, with minimal stress on joints and ligaments, your muscles will feel like they've had a real workout! You will feel energized and achieve faster muscle definition in less time than using conventional weights. Even those with asthma and fibromyalgia can achieve weight loss and toning results.

The Science behind Revolutionary Vibration Plate Machine Technology

Hundreds of studies, including those of *NASA*, highlight the many positive benefits of whole body vibration, revealing that it can achieve results in a much shorter period than conventional or even more intensive training methods. Astronauts use this therapy to quickly build lost muscle and bone mass after their space missions. Many chiropractors recommend vibration plates to help prevent bone loss and osteoporosis. Many physicians recommend it to help balance hormones after child birth and during all stages of menopause.

Achieve FAST RESULTS with a minimum of effort. It you want more toned, defined muscles, a lifted and firm butt, flat abs, or a smaller waist and hips - it's not quantity you need- just a better quality muscle workout provided by Vibration Plate Technology. A Body Vibration Plate can:

-increase muscle strength up to 50% in as little as three weeks;
-help prevent bone mineral loss;
-prevent osteoporosis and help build bone density;
-help speed fat burning;
-sculpt, tone and define muscles far FASTER than most other conventional exercises;
-reduce muffin tops and inches around the waist;
-quickly tone the stomach and core muscles FASTER than doing crunches or sit-ups;
-reshape the arms, hips, waist, abdomen and legs;
-help tighten skin on the body, face. It even helps tone facial muscles;
-reduce and smooth dimply cellulite by enhancing collagen production;
-promote lymphatic drainage to improve the skin's texture and tone;
-increase human growth hormone (HGH) output by up to 361% to help rejuvenate the body;
-offer a safe and far less costly option to HGH injections;
-enhance metabolic rate and increase energy;
-reduce stress and decrease cortisol production (stress hormone) to help eliminate middle-aged spread;
-help uplift mood and sense of wellbeing;
-help balance hormones whether post-baby, PMS, or menopause;
-reduce menopausal issues such as irritability, mood swings, hot flashes and night sweats;
-reduce insomnia and increase libido;
-offer a workout alternative for everyone including those with fibromyalgia or asthma;
-offer a home workout for stay-at-home moms and busy women on the go;
-promote blood circulation and help strengthen the immune system; and
-increase joint mobility.

How Do I Use A Body Vibration Plate?

Stand, sit or lay on the vibration plate to perform several different body toning exercises. Below are a variety of poses and exercises to choose from. To speed results, I recommend performing 10 positions in the morning and 10 at night. You can also perform 20 or 30 positions in a 20 or 30 minute session. I recommend the 30 minute workout for those who are accustomed to working out. See some very effective poses and exercises below.

NOTE: Be sure to drink a big glass of water before and after each session.

*Stand on the plate with knees slightly bent, while holding the arm straps up. Tightly squeeze the bicep muscles of the arms for 60 seconds. Watch the timer on the LCD screen. After 60 seconds, move to the next position. NOTE: Engage the stomach muscles while holding all the positions and exercises noted for faster tummy toning.

*Stand with knees slightly bent and do a pelvic tilt while holding and squeezing the buttock muscles tightly for 60 seconds.

*Hold a deep squat position and squeeze thigh muscles for 60 seconds.

*Stand with feet hip width apart and stand on toes, squeeze calves, legs, butt and hold tummy in at the same time for 60 seconds.

*Stand with feet hip width apart and balance on heels. Squeeze buttocks and thighs and hold tummy in at the same time for 60 seconds.

*Step off the plate and hold a lunge with one leg resting on the vibration plate, holding the lunge for 60 seconds. Repeat the lunge position on the other leg, squeezing and holding for 60 seconds.

*Sit on the vibration plate with legs straddled apart, toes pointed, and squeeze leg muscles tightly. This helps reduce cellulite on back of thighs and tones the legs quickly. Engage stomach and sit tall. This reduces the 'muffin tops' within two to three weeks.

*Roll onto one side of the thigh and squeeze for 60 seconds. This addresses cellulite/saddle bag areas. Roll onto the other side of the thigh and repeat.

*Hold an abdominal crunch pose for even faster tummy toning results.

*Sit on the plate and cross legs, holding a lotus pose for 60 seconds.

*To perform the super gal pose, lie with your tummy on the plate with legs and arms extended, toes and fingers pointed, and squeeze butt and legs for 60 seconds.

*Hold a push-up position and feel the vibrations up the arms, down the back and down to the tummy. Hold stomach in while doing this exercise too.

*For those who are more advanced, hold a plank position on one arm for 60 seconds. Repeat on the other side.

*Do a series of 20 push-ups (or more).

*Do a series of 60 squats (or more).

Many positions can be performed on a vibration plate, so you'll never be bored. As you get stronger, incorporate more gym exercises on your plate or increase the time to 20 minutes. See more exercises in the user manual.

Workout in your PJs

I urge women to get out of bed, and while in their PJs, sit or stand on the vibration plate for just 10 minutes in the morning. It's a great way to start the day - especially if you have a high stress schedule; you're a new mom wishing to get into shape; or if going through hormonal changes such as menopause. A **Body Vibration Plate** uplifts your mood, triggers fat burning and much more.

Women and men everywhere, from moms and dads to actresses, models, athletes, and busy baby boomers, are discovering that using a body vibration machine in the privacy of their own home is the answer they've been waiting for. It's a more convenient and faster way to help achieve weight loss and a toned, firm, rejuvenated body - just 10 minutes a day!

NOTE: Check with your healthcare practitioner before ordering this item.

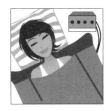

Age-Proofing Tip #59
FIR Infrared Sauna Blanket For
Rapid Weight Loss & Wellbeing

NOTE: As always, consult a physician or medical professional before beginning a heat therapy regimen to see if you are physically capable and can undergo such treatment without serious consequence.

I'm excited to introduce the FIR infrared sauna blanket, as an affordable alternative health, beauty, and weight loss home and professional treatment. I've shared this therapy with many women since 2011. Several health experts, hormone doctors and Dr. Oz himself promote the weight loss, health and wellbeing benefits of FIR infrared sauna therapy.

Traditional sauna heat is not absorbed by the body. It simply makes us sweat water. FIR infrared sauna heat, on the other hand, is absorbed by the cells which dilates them, resulting in better blood circulation, oxygenation and an overall improved metabolism. Regular use of an FIR infrared sauna blanket is an effective addition to regular exercise for cardiovascular conditioning and burning of calories. You can burn up to 600 calories in just one hour. FIR infrared heat speeds lipolysis to help reduce unwanted fat in tummy, waist, buttocks, hips, arms, and legs. Infrared heat is recommended by fitness experts because it can help reduce the stubborn middle bulge. In fact, many hours after a treatment the body continues to burn calories. This blanket is used in detox and weight loss clinics nationwide.

FIR (Far Infrared Radiation) heat is not only safe and comfortable; it provides benefits that conventional saunas can't. From improved skin texture and lower blood pressure, to soothed joints, relief of stiff or sore muscles infrared heat is outstanding for all women and men.

In addition, the circulation provided by FIR heat can help remove toxic chemicals from muscles and organs, and induces relaxation and a feeling of wellbeing, providing significant psychological as well as physiological benefits. It even helps improve sleep.

More Benefits of FIR Infrared Sauna Blankets

*Infrared therapy has proven to be effective because its 'hot rays' offer analgesic, anti-inflammatory relief.

*Increases heart rate and blood circulation <u>without raising blood pressure</u>, both of which are crucial to maintaining our health. The heart rate increases as blood flow diverts away from the inner organs towards the extremities of the skin. The increased flow helps aching or injured muscles recover faster, and speeds the removal of toxic waste from the body through skin perspiration. The skin helps eliminate up to 30% of body waste. As noted in Dr. Alicia Stanton's popular book, *The Complete Idiots Guide to Hormone Weight Loss*, "As much as 15% of the sweat produced is composed of dissolved toxins.... they are an excellent way to reduce stress and toxins. These key factors can reduce cortisol demand, which triggers weight loss and keeps hormones balanced."

*Used in detox and health clinics nationwide. Women experiencing hormonal changes find them helpful for clearing toxins, fat burning and relieving soreness. An article in *Healthy Living* revealed that Suzanne Somers credits her continued good health to regular use of infrared heat to help eliminate and sweat out heavy metals. Many wellness experts advocate using infrared heat therapy for detoxification. It is a gentle approach to removing chemical toxins. A study presented at the *2012 Biological Medicine Conference* found that "the perspiration of people using a conventional sauna was 95-97% water, while the perspiration of those using infrared saunas was just 80-85% percent water and the non-water elimination contained fat-soluble toxins, heavy metals, sulfuric acid, sodium, ammonia and uric acid."

*Heat and high calorie-burning sweat aids in weight loss by speeding up the metabolic process of vital organs and endocrine glands resulting in a substantial caloric loss.

*For a healthy 'glow,' FIR infrared sauna therapy allows increased blood circulation to carry great amounts of nutrients to the skin, resulting in smoother, healthier-looking skin.

*FIR infrared heat helps increase the immune system by creating an 'artificial fever.' A fever is the natural healing response of the body which aids the immune system to naturally ward off viral and bacterial growth, and other invading organisms. Incorporating a FIR heat treatment, during the beginning signs of a cold or flu, can help prevent and even stop the progression of full blown symptoms. Even further studies of FIR heat therapy have created a buzz for those challenged with life threatening diseases such as cancer. See more on use to aid cancer treatment below.

*Cancer patients and survivors use infrared heat therapy to remove chemical toxins. Recent studies reveal that heat therapy, along with chemotherapy and other cancer treatments, can offer many health benefits for cancer patients. Tumor cells are affected by the high temperatures reached by infrared sauna heat and can 'weaken' cancerous cells. FIR heat can enhance chemo or radiation therapy that may help reduce the number of treatments or drug dosage required, which can uplift the cancer patient both mentally and physcially.

*FIR infrared heat is used in the medical and holistic communities and as medical treatment performed by doctors, chiropractors, acupuncturists, physical therapists, detox centers, weight loss clinics, trainers, massage therapists, fitness enthusiasts and athletes. FIR infrared sauna blankets can help those challenged with arthritis, joint pain, stiff muscles, fibromyalgia, injuries to tendons and ligaments, to promote faster self-healing and even weight loss.

*Having a FIR infrared treatment before a massage reduces stress and instills relaxation. It loosens the muscle tissue so the therapist can perform a more thorough and effective massage.

The Science behind FIR Infrared Sauna Heat

Unlike visible light, FIR infrared sauna heat deeply penetrates skin and underlying tissues (over 1 ½"). Infrared energy naturally generates heat by causing the body's molecules to rapidly vibrate against each other. When infrared rays penetrate the skin, they come into contact with protein, collagen and fats, and cause a thermal reaction which raises the tissue temperatures. The human body then reacts by dilating all the blood vessels regardless of size. Tissues are revitalized as a result of improved circulation.

One of the main principles of traditional Chinese medicine is that good blood circulation promotes good health. They believe that slow blood flow may increase the likelihood of disease and pain.

NOTE: For adults aged 18 and up. If you have any health concerns, check with your healthcare practitioner before purchasing this item.

Regular FIR infrared sauna blanket treatments can provide the following benefits:

-improve the immune system;
-reduce inflammation and pain;
-help remedy sleeping disorders;
-detoxify the body and burn fat quickly and safely;
-promote the excretion of heavy metals, toxins, and other waste deposits in the body;
-help speed metabolism and enhance absorption of nutrients;
-offer a health and wellbeing option for patients of physical therapists, doctors, detox, weight loss and cancer centers; and
-benefit athletes and sports enthusiasts to reduce sore muscles.

Go to www.BeautyLifechanger.com for more information.

Specifications include:

-XXL size with overall dimensions: 72" x 36" x 2" thickness. There is no height limit;
-3 zones of infrared heating therapy for upper, middle or lower body or all three areas simultaneously. Each zone includes manual temperature selection;
-temperature reaches up to 167 degrees Fahrenheit (85 degrees Celsius);
-60 minute timer! Reset timer for longer sessions;
-one year warranty for parts and repairs;
-used by adults ages 18 and up; and
-use in any 110v outlet.

NOTE: Check with your doctor before ordering this item and if you have any health concerns.

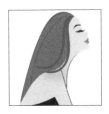

Age-Proofing Tip #60
Fabulous Hair Tips

For healthy, lustrous hair, consume foods that are rich in protein and healthy oils including essential omega 3 fatty acids found in flaxseed oil, avocados, and fish such as wild salmon, tuna or sardines. Other excellent oils for hair are plant-based omega 6s and 9s such as olive, coconut, safflower, evening primrose, walnut and pumpkin oil. Hair-healthy nuts include almonds, walnuts, pistachios and pumpkin seeds. Also include a variety of vitamin and mineral-rich vegetables and low-glycemic fruits to enhance the growth and condition of your hair. **NOTE:** Check with your doctor before taking supplements noted.

*An excellent green food supplement called chlorella, softens and adds shine to hair. In addition, it improves skin, nails and uplifts our mood. Chlorella is an immune-boosting green food that offers even more age-proofing benefits. Chlorella is formulated into powerful pellets that can be taken after meals or placed into a morning protein smoothie. Read many more benefits of chlorella in **Age-Proofing Tip #51 - My Favorite Supplements for Women.**

*As noted on earlier pages, hyaluronic acid (HA) is highly beneficial for hydrating the skin, eyes, lips and joints. In addition, HA moisturizes the deep layers of the scalp, which can prevent thinning and falling hair. HA can be taken as an oral supplement.

*Below is an excellent scalp hydrating recipe recommended by top hair stylist, Mary Jo Lorie. **Here's what you do:**

Lightly scrape the scalp using a comb. Hold it at a 45-degree angle, gently pushing the comb back and forth to loosen dead skin cells. Then mix 2 tbsp. vitamin E oil with 2 tbsp. almond or olive oil. Warm the oils in the microwave for 10 seconds or use at room temperature. Section the hair about ½" apart. Apply the oil mixture on scalp using a dropper. Place a shower cap over hair. Leave on for one hour or overnight. Then shampoo hair as normal.

*Many women are low in zinc and iron which can cause thinning hair, female pattern baldness, brittle or weak nails and depression. These key trace minerals address many body functions that support healthy follicles, hair and nail growth, calm inflammation, keep acne in check, and uplift mood. In addition, low levels of zinc can cause slow wound healing and increase body odor. Read label directions for dosage.

*To stimulate hair growth, prevent hair loss and add body to hair, choose shampoos that moisturize the scalp and are free of parabens, synthetic fragrances and sodium laurel sulfates (SLS). Sodium lauryl sulfates fade hair color and strip away natural scalp oils causing dull, dry or brittle hair. SLS can even damage and dry the scalp which can result in thinning, falling hair. I noted two very effective and well-priced SLS-free brands below:

For those with thinning or falling hair, my current favorite shampoo and conditioning products are made by **Your Crown & Glory** (YC&G). Their products are organic, non-toxic, and free of SLSs, 1-4 Dioxane, parabens or phthalates. Formulated with apple juice, natural extracts, and B vitamins, this line of well-priced products will not strip hair color and addresses thinning, falling hair concerns. YC&G manufacturers formulated **Lavender Shampoo** for women, **Lemon Shampoo** for men, and a popular, universal **Peppermint Conditioner**. They also formulated a **Walnut Shampoo** (scalp scrub) to unplug hair follicles and aid hair growth. The light lather cleans, adds body, luster, strength and hydration to hair and scalp. YC&G is for all hair types - normal, dry, coarse, thinning or falling hair, and those challenged with eczema or psoriasis on the scalp. The frequent comment I receive from those who use these products is that their hair has more body and shine. Elle Magazine voted **Your Crown & Glory Conditioner** as a favorite.

*For limp, lifeless hair, another excellent brand of hair products is **Giovanni® Root 66™ Max Volume Shampoo** and **Conditioner**. Giovanni® hair products are organic, SLS-free with natural scents and free of parabens and phthalates. See more paraben and phthalate-free hair products choices in **Safe & Effective Face & Body Product Suggestions.**

*Teasing the crown of the hair can add volume to limp, thin hair. To naturally increase volume, massage a little cornstarch onto the hair at the crown of the scalp. **Here's what you do:**

Lift up sections of the hair on the crown area and massage about ½ tsp. cornstarch into the roots of the hair. Then tease hair 3-4" from the scalp down.

*For those with gray hair, I've read several reports that unsulphured molasses may help reverse grayness. Consuming 1 tbsp. of molasses per day is recommended. Add it to hot tea or oatmeal. I've noted a tasty oatmeal recipe for two below. **Here's what you do:**

Combine 1 cup water with ½ cup steel cut oats, a pinch of salt, and bring to a boil. Turn heat down and add ¼ tsp. cinnamon, ½ sliced banana, 1 tsp. ground flax meal, 1 tbsp. unsulphured blackstrap molasses and 4 tbsp. rice, soy, or almond milk. Stir ingredients and simmer with lid slightly ajar for 17-18 minutes. Yummy!

*Always use conditioner on ends of hair and use cool water as a final rinse. This closes hair follicles and adds shine.

*For those with dry or color processed hair, make a hair hydrating mask once a week. **Here's what you do:**

Massage 2-3 tbsp. argan oil on scalp and hair from roots to ends. Leave on overnight. In the morning, shampoo and condition hair as usual and you'll be left with shiny hair with body.

*Do not scrunch or rub hair with a towel after washing as this creates tangles and makes combing more difficult. Instead, very gently squeeze out excess water and wrap hair in a towel.

*Use a wide-toothed comb or fingers to gently comb through wet hair. The best way to comb out long, wet, tangled hair is by starting at the ends and working your way up.

*For those with curly hair, scrunch some pure aloe vera gel onto wet curls to eliminate frizzies all day long.

*Before blow drying, apply a protein-infused product to protect hair.

*Use a medium heat setting to blow dry hair. **Here's what you do:**

Hold dryer four to six inches away from hair to prevent damage. Finish drying with a blast of cool air to close hair follicles and add shine. Invest in an ion blow dryer. The ions in the warm air break down water molecules and lock in moisture. Ion dryers dry hair faster, preventing dry, frizzy or damaged hair.

*Don't have time to shampoo? Use coconut flour to make a natural dry shampoo alternative. Coconut flour absorbs oil. **Here's what you do:**

Place 1 tsp. coconut flour in a little bowl. Lift up sections of the hair and massage the flour into the scalp and roots. Wait three minutes and brush through hair.

*If you don't have coconut flour, combine cornstarch and baking soda to make this alternate dry shampoo recipe. **Here's what you do:**

Combine 1 tsp. cornstarch and ½ tsp. baking soda. Separate sections of the hair and massage the powder into scalp and roots. Then brush through hair. Baking soda removes odors and cornstarch soaks up oils for a temporary and safe hair cleaning alternative.

*My conditioning hair pak is an effective monthly treatment for those with chemically processed or dry hair. **Here's what you do:**

Combine ½ mashed avocado, 1 slightly beaten egg and 2 tbsp. olive or safflower oil. Shampoo hair and apply mixture on wet, clean hair. Put on a shower cap. To boost penetration, warm a towel in the dryer and wrap the warm towel over the shower cap. Leave on for 30 minutes. Shampoo hair again and condition as normal.

Reverse Thinning, Falling Hair

Hair Loss Facts
*50% of men and women experience significant hair loss.
*60% of menopausal women experience thinning hair.
*The average person loses 50-100 hairs per day.

*There are many reasons for thinning or falling hair including hormonal imbalances, thyroid issues, improper nutrition, product buildup, and stress. If experiencing thinning or falling hair increase shampooing hair to at least three times a week. Why? Environmental pollutants, natural scalp oils, perspiration, and styling products can harden and trap the hair follicles. This causes hair to break off, hindering hair growth.

*The function of the follicle is to protect and hold hair in the scalp as it grows. Each follicle holds one or two hairs. At the base of each follicle, there is an opening called the papilla which produces new hair growth. The quality of the hair produced by the papilla relies on circulation, hydration and a healthy diet. Consume a variety of colorful fruits and vegetables, healthy oils, and B vitamins, including B-12 (sublingual supplements).

*If experiencing sudden hair loss, you may be low in the mineral zinc or have a thyroid imbalance. Other signs of zinc deficiency are depression, low energy, frequent colds, brain fog, strong body odor and acne breakouts.

*To prevent thinning hair, consume foods such as healthy omega 3, 6 and 9 fatty acids found in coconut, safflower, evening primrose, walnut, flaxseed and pumpkin oil. Good protein choices for healthy hair are fresh fish such as salmon or tuna; nuts such as almonds, walnuts, pistachios and pumpkin seeds. In addition, include a variety of colorful vegetables and low-glycemic fruits in your diet.

Is Hair Loss Hereditary?

*Hair loss is not hereditary. However, the number of sweat and oil glands on the scalp are hereditary. The higher the number of glands, the higher incidence of hair loss.

*Men naturally produce more oil and perspiration than women do, resulting in more trapped follicles and falling hair.

*Both women and men produce the hormone testosterone. The amount of testosterone in our bodies plays a role in hair loss. When an enzyme called 5 alpha-reductase increases, it converts testosterone into DHT (dihydrotestosterone). The DHT remains in the scalp's follicles which clogs and cuts off nutrition to the hair, causing it to fall. The excess of DHT is the main cause of thinning, falling hair in both women and men. Production of DHT can be hereditary or a result of hormone imbalances in both men and women. Choose hair products that can help balance the DHT on the scalp, such as YC&G noted at the top of this section. They help unplug the trapped hair follicles, increase blood flow, promote hair growth, and hydrate and nourish the scalp and follicles.

*Keeping the scalp clean can help prevent a clogged scalp. To remove product buildup from hair and scalp, this easy recipe is fast and effective. **Here's what you do:**

Combine 1 tbsp. baking soda with shampoo and massage into wet hair and scalp.Then rinse and condition hair as usual.

*My scalp hydrating tonic is healthy and easy to make. **Here's what you do:**

Steep 2 peppermint tea bags in ¼ cup of boiled water for 10 minutes. Remove bags and allow tea to cool to room temperature. Add 2 tbsp. olive oil and 1 tbsp. eucalyptus oil and stir. Wash hair and massage the scalp hydrator onto scalp. Put on a plastic shower cap and leave on for 30 minutes. Afterward, shampoo and condition hair as usual.

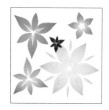

More Empowering Tips

Jump into Life – Do Something Fearless

We work to pay our bills, put food on our tables, and provide for our families. But after work, how we spend time is ultimately our choice. So why not take the opportunity to try new and fun things? Some of us are so overwhelmed with work and responsibilities that somewhere along the way we forget to 'stop and smell the roses.' We've stopped having fun.

Has your day to day life become routine? Does it sound like this? You work, come home, cook, eat, clean up, do some laundry, watch TV, and then go to sleep. On weekends, you run errands and do housework. Don't get me wrong. Some individuals enjoy this type of routine so that's a good thing. But for those who feel restless, bored or have lost their zest for life, maybe it's time to try something fearless.

"'I can't do it' - never yet accomplished anything; 'I will try' - has performed wonders." – George P. Burnham

Pick three things you would like to try. Perhaps take a lesson in trapeze, ballroom or pole dancing (a great workout too). If you're more adventurous, try hang-gliding or scuba diving. If you're not into those types of activities, go to a rock concert on a weeknight. You can handle a late night every once in a while, right? Perhaps plan a little weekend road trip for some wine tasting adventures, and visit local museums and art fairs. Who knows? You may be inspired to take up a new hobby like painting or drawing.

If life feels dull and routine, try something to spice it up. Do something you would never dream of doing otherwise. I'm not talking about doing something illegal or dishonest. For example, do you dream of singing or playing piano? Then why not invest in singing or piano lessons? Who knows - you may just be the next big discovery on 'The X Factor' or 'America's Got Talent!' They've discovered talent of all ages. Remember the now famous singer, Susan Boyle?

"What you do today can change the course of your entire life far into the future. Today is critical. Today really counts." – Ralph S. Marston, Jr.

Perhaps you're afraid to speak in front of people. I myself once had this fear only seven or eight years ago. It was moments before my first appearance on a television show as an author and beauty expert. I had done 100s of radio interviews but being on a live TV show was new for me. As I waited for my introduction, my throat felt glued shut and I began to panic. Luckily, I gulped down some water and took a moment to say a prayer and had a little 'talk' with myself. I knew in my heart that what I was about to share with my viewers would be information they would want. Sure enough, as I stepped in front of the cameras, I felt an immediate calmness rush through me. The fear *instantly* left my body and I felt excited and overjoyed. I was 'in my element' and my segment turned out to be a hit! In fact, I was invited back to share more tips. The positive experience and feedback built up my confidence and set the wheels in motion for even bigger opportunities to come my way. Since that time, I've done countless television appearances and to this day, I still get a mixed rush of excitement and calmness when I'm on TV.

Discover your unlimited potential. Approach each day with a sense of adventure. Once you jump into life, family, friends and co-workers will want to know your secret. You may just find yourself becoming a role model for others. Is today the day you choose to make a new beginning? Be prepared to see your life transform in all areas. Know it and own it! Now go out there and be fearless. ☺

"Leap and the net will appear." – Julie Cameron

Acknowledge Others

Be mindful to acknowledge others along your life's path. The expression, 'smile and the world smiles with you' is so true! Some individuals embrace life, choosing to walk their daily path as if a ray of sunshine is upon them. Others carry a scowl on their faces, as if walking under a dark cloud. Perhaps they're dealing with a trauma or challenging situation. We cannot judge. For the majority of us, though, a smile can improve how we feel.

Many studies have proven that smiling can instantly uplift us. Try smiling now! ☺ Powerful, isn't it? One study noted that a smiling person standing in a crowded room attracts <u>twice</u> as much attention. Another benefit of smiling is that it's age-proofing. It lifts a sagging jaw line and jowls - like a mini-face-lift. Look in the mirror and smile. See what I mean? Ta-daaa! No more droopy jowls.

"Most people are about as happy as they make their minds up to be."
– Abraham Lincoln

Embrace Life's Challenges

As noted earlier, it's important to begin each day with a positive attitude. Of course, we can't expect to be feeling up 24/7. That's not realistic. There are going to be some tough situations in life that we will all face at some time. It's a part of life. As we create our lives one day at a time, it's perfectly healthy to have a good cry or to feel angry when we experience tough situations such as the loss of a loved one or your job, or a break up. However, it's what we do after a reasonable amount of time grieving, that we can learn and grow from.

Pamper and heal yourself and try not to dwell for too long. Embrace the lesson learned and you will quickly triumph over it. Life's challenges may help us find the courage to face situations we've ignored. They may help us become more grateful, compassionate or self-sufficient. Who knows? Maybe this 'bump in the road' will motivate you to go after your dreams. Embracing and overcoming life's challenges empowers us. Nothing can stand between you and your happiness.

"There's only one thing more painful than learning from experience, and that is not learning from experience." – Laurence J. Peter

If not able to move past a 'trapped state' (experiencing hopelessness, low energy, panic attacks, thoughts of suicide or feel depressed) you may be challenged with thyroid changes, adrenal exhaustion or hormonal imbalance. Be sure to seek the advice of a healthcare practitioner. We are each worthy of a fulfilling and happy life, success and good health. ☺

Give Back

"To measure the man, measure his heart." – Malcolm Stevenson Forbes

Volunteering a little time each week or month can make a positive difference in your life and the lives of others too. Visit your local children's hospital or retirement home and read books to those in need.

If you like animals, why not help out at an animal shelter? Who knows - while volunteering, you may just find Mr. Right standing next to you. You'll know that his heart is in the right place too.

Giving blood is another excellent way to give back. Just 45 minutes of your time and a pint of blood can save three lives! If you're a busy individual, send a check to the Red Cross or your favorite charity or cause.

Another way to give back is by performing a random act of kindness. Offer iced tea to your delivery person or buy a cup of coffee for a person standing in line behind you at a coffee shop. Give your friend a little gift or some flowers even when it's not her birthday. Often the greatest gift you can give someone is to take time to listen. These thoughtful acts of kindness can uplift you too.

Enjoy Good Food & an Occasional Sinful Treat

Eating is a big part of living life. Excessive dieting and deprivation isn't fun or healthy. I know this from experience. At the beginning of my modeling career, I practically starved myself to stay at 115 pounds and a size four. I looked lean and mean, I counted calories, and like many models, I also took laxatives. Luckily, after about two years of this unhealthy behavior, I sought counseling with an eating disorder specialist. He helped me address this challenge, after just three sessions.

According to the Renfrew Center Foundation for Eating Disorders almost 24 million people in the United States suffer from eating disorders. An article in USA Today noted that 47% of middle school and high-school aged girls go on diets because of the photos they see in magazines.

Rather than dieting, I stick to eating healthy, delicious foods including a variety of pesticide-free vegetables, low-glycemic fruits and hormone and antibiotic-free protein products - six days a week. Then once a week, my husband and I will enjoy a cheat day where we indulge in a few french fries, pasta or a veggie pizza. On special occasions, such as birthdays and anniversaries, we'll have decadent dinner out and then split a piece of carrot cake or another sinful treat. Prior to having a special meal, I take my doctor-approved 'Slimming Tonic' noted in **Age-Proofing Tip #56 - Boost Your Metabolism.**

Camouflaging Extra Inches

Enjoying holiday desserts and cocktails usually results in a few extra pounds and inches. No worries! Until you get back to your comfortable weight, a great way to hide extra inches is to invest in a waist-cinching undergarment. I like the **Underscore®** brand at JC Penney because it provides better waist cinching support than *that* famous brand many celebrities wear on the red carpet. Plus the Underscore® is under $30. Even while carrying a few extra pounds, I try not to be too hard on myself. In fact, my weight hovers around 132 pounds and since I no longer feel the pressure to be bone thin, I am much happier and healthier. Plus my husband seems to be enjoying my curves - even after all these years together. Hee hee.

Daily Advice for Every Woman

A colleague of mine, Stephanie de Phillipo, is a professional health and fitness expert dedicated to integrated holistic living. She is a life counselor, yoga therapist, nutritionist for natural health and immunity, and is the creator of 'Tantric Toning' Mind/Body Program and DVD that is the answer to fitness for women. Stephanie is a writer, has been featured in L.A Magazine, Women's Wear Daily, and is a graduate of the Wharton School. Find out more about Stephanie at StephaniesSacredSelfCare.com and enjoy some of her favorite tips for women below:

*Remind yourself how blessed your life is. Don't sink into thoughts about what you 'should' be doing. You're doing it. If lower thoughts arise just notice them, recognize and change them into positives. Take care of how you think.

*Don't just work to the point of having no free time. Become more involved with friends, or join a group and meet with them once a week.

*Do something artistic with beads, paint, collages, or maybe dedicate a beautiful altar to your beautiful self. You'll see it daily, as an honor to you. Reflect on all your goodness, you goddesses!

*Smile at yourself in the mirror and see how great you look. Smile into your eyes and appreciate that loving face of yours. See your graceful beauty.

*Eat a delicious meal. Enjoy a glass of wine to satisfy and relax yourself, improve digestion and just plain enjoy really stimulating your palette. Eat slowly. No rushing. Just enjoy every bite.

*Think like a child. Let things be simple whenever you can and watch life unfold as it gets simpler.

*Relish in self-care. Attend to yourself especially after enjoying a soothing bath. Use your loving, gentle hands to apply healthy creams and serums onto your skin. Notice all your body parts and how they feel and look.

*Play your favorite songs that formed your teens and dance with all your heart. (Don't forget to shake your booty.)

*Ask yourself, "Do I give enough? Do I do enough? Do I rise to the occasion?"

*Live in the present. Focus on what you're doing now. Learn not to focus on the past and you'll move forward - like never before.

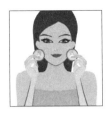

More Beauty Recipes

In addition to beauty recipes noted on earlier pages, I have noted more of my favorite beauty recipes below. Please do not use any of these tips/home remedies if you are allergic to the ingredients noted. The recipes noted are for all skin types, unless otherwise noted. These recipes are not meant to replace diagnosis by a health professional or cure any disease. Readers assume all risk with use or misuse of the recipes and suggestions.

Facial Beauty Recipes for all skin types (unless otherwise noted)

Facial Moisturizer for All Skin Types

Ingredients:
6 tbsp. squalane oil (from olives)
3 tbsp. jojoba oil

Combine the oils to make an exceptional facial moisturizer for all skin types. Squalane oil is similar to the skin's natural sebum and helps stimulate collagen. Jojoba oil is rich in anti-aging vitamin E. Apply after cleansing and toning the skin.

Turmeric Skin Brightener Mask

For those challenged with sensitive skin with age spots, antioxidant-rich turmeric (a spice) contains anti-inflammatory properties that can help calm sensitive skin and fade spots. Honey is a natural hydrator and antibacterial, and yogurt helps brighten skin.

Ingredients:
¼ tsp. turmeric
1 tbsp. honey
1 tbsp. plain yogurt

Combine turmeric, honey and yogurt. Apply on clean skin and leave on for 30 minutes. Rinse skin with tepid water and pat skin dry. Apply your favorite moisturizer.

Apple Age Spot Reducer (not for those with rosacea)

Malic acid in apples, lemon juice and turmeric are highly effective skin lighteners and brighteners. Apples are rich in vitamins A, B, C, K, biotin and pantothenic acid and provide skin rejuvenating benefits. Lemons contain citric acid which naturally bleaches skin. Turmeric is an antioxidant-rich spice that also offers anti-inflammatory benefits to calm the redness associated with rosacea. Honey hydrates and calms the skin and is a natural antibacterial. To reduce age spots, melasma and fine lines, this recipe is beneficial.

Ingredients:
1 raw, peeled and cored apple
2 tbsp. honey
2 tsp. fresh lemon juice
¼ tsp. turmeric

Place apple in a blender or food processor until finely chopped. Transfer to a bowl, add remainder of the ingredients and mix well. Apply on clean skin and leave on for 30 minutes.

Brown Sugar Spot Fader
(not for those with rosacea)

Try this mask weekly to help fade pigmentation spots.

Ingredients:
3 tbsp. brown sugar
1 tbsp. raw honey
1 tbsp. fresh lemon juice

Combine the ingredients in a small bowl. Apply mixture on clean skin, focusing on the pigmented areas and scrub for 30 seconds. Then, scrub entire face and leave on for three to five minutes. Rinse off with tepid water. Mixture lasts three days in the refrigerator.

Witch Hazel & Lemon Spot Reducer
(not for those with rosacea)

After using the following recipe for just 18 days, one of my readers was so delighted with her results, she sent before and after photos! See her photos on the LED Red Light Therapy page at www.hollywoodbeautysecrets.com

Ingredients:
½ lemon juice (freshly squeezed, not bottled)
3 oz. witch hazel

Combine the ingredients to make a natural bleaching toner. Apply on pigmented areas using a cotton ball or swab nightly. After three weeks spots will be faded. Keep refrigerated up to four days, then discard and make a fresh batch.

Exfoliating Masks for All Skin Types (unless otherwise noted)

Pumpkin Enzyme Peel Exfoliator

Pumpkin is a <u>fruit</u> that is rich in carotene, vitamins A, C and E, as well as skin healing enzymes that gently exfoliate skin, unclog pores and smooth fine lines.

Ingredients:
3 tbsp. plain, canned pumpkin
1 tsp. honey
1 tsp. milk or cream

Combine ingredients in a glass bowl and stir to a paste. Apply on clean skin and leave on for 20 minutes. Rinse the mask off with tepid water.

Papaya Enzyme Peel

The enzymes in papaya gently exfoliate skin, repair sun damage, diminish pigmentation spots and help brighten and smooth skin. It's a natural alternative to Retin-A®.

Once a week, cut a papaya in half. Scoop out the seeds and pulp. Eat the pulp - it's great for digestion and tastes delicious. Rub the inside of the peel of the papaya on clean face, under eyes, on lips and neck. Wait 20 minutes or until the mask dries. Rinse with tepid water.

Jojoba Oil & Corn Meal Scrub (not for those with rosacea)

Ingredients:

1 tbsp. jojoba oil
1 tbsp. plain yogurt (or Half and Half®)
1 tbsp. baking soda
1 tsp. corn meal

Combine oil, yogurt (or Half and Half®), baking soda and corn meal to make an effective scrub. Apply on clean skin and scrub in a gentle circular motion; rinse and pat skin dry.

Glycerin, Sea Salt & Baking Soda Scrub (not for those with rosacea)

Ingredients:
2 tbsp. vegetable glycerin
1 tbsp. sea salt
1 tbsp. baking soda

Combine ingredients in a small bowl and stir to a paste. Apply on clean skin and scrub face and neck in a gentle, circular motion. Rinse off with tepid water and pat skin dry.

Powdered Milk & Honey Mask (not for those with rosacea)

Ingredients:
3 tbsp. powdered milk
2 tbsp. honey

Combine ingredients in a small bowl and stir to a paste. Apply on clean skin and scrub face and neck in gentle circular motion. Rinse off with tepid water and pat skin dry.

Coconut Oil Exfoliating Mask

Ingredients:
½ tsp. coconut oil (organic food grade)

Food grade coconut oil rejuvenates and hydrates all skin types, fades wrinkles, sun spots, scars and prevents acne/blemish breakouts! This non-pore-clogging oil gently exfoliates skin and strengthens underlying tissues. It helps smooth lines and hydrates all skin types. It's rich in caprylic acid which keeps acne/blemishes in check too. Coconut oil absorbs into the skin's cells and helps fight free radical damage associated with sun exposure.

Apply this recipe before bedtime. Run a metal spoon under hot water. While the spoon is still warm, scoop about ½ tsp. coconut oil from the jar onto clean fingertips. The solid coconut oil will easily melt on fingertips as you spread it *sparingly* on clean skin.

Soothing, Hydrating Masks for All Skin Types (unless otherwise noted)

Egg & Honey Facial Mask

Honey is a natural humectant and antibacterial, eggs help brighten skin and reduce sun spots, while the avocado contains natural omega 3 fatty acids to help moisturize all skin types.

Ingredients:
1 egg yolk
1 tbsp. honey
2 tbsp. avocado

Combine egg yolk, honey and avocado in a small bowl. Apply mask to clean skin and leave on for 20 minutes. Rinse off with tepid water.

Wrinkle Reducer & Face Rejuvenator

This fast and easy beauty recipe helps hydrate and soften skin, reduces the appearance of wrinkles and alleviates chapped, cracked or rough winter skin. Honey is a natural hydrator and antibacterial.

Ingredients:
1 powder capsule CoQ10
1 tsp. honey

Open CoQ10 capsule and pour into honey. After cleansing, apply the mixture on clean face, around eyes and on neck. After 45 minutes rinse skin with tepid water and pat skin dry.

Rosacea Redness Reducing Mask

For those challenged with red, sensitive skin associated with rosacea, antioxidant-rich turmeric (a spice) contains anti-inflammatory properties that can help calm redness. Honey is a natural hydrator and antibacterial.

Ingredients:
¼ tsp. turmeric
2 tbsp. honey

Combine ingredients and apply on clean skin. Leave on for 30 minutes. Rinse with tepid water.

Sunburned Skin Calmer Mask

Vitamin A and enzymes in pumpkin provide skin healing properties, reduce redness, gently exfoliate and speed skin healing. Honey is a humectant that hydrates, contains natural antibiotic properties that heal skin and antibacterial agents that clean skin.

Ingredients:
2 tbsp. plain, canned pumpkin
1 tsp. honey

Combine pumpkin and honey. Apply mask on clean skin. Leave on for 15 minutes and then rinse with tepid water.

Potato Skin Firmer
(mature skin)

This facial mask rejuvenates and firms mature, sagging skin. Potatoes are rich in vitamin C, B6, potassium, manganese, fiber and tryptophan. The starch in potatoes creates a skin firming affect.

Ingredients:
½ cooked, mashed potato
1 egg yolk
1 tsp. cream

Combine the ingredients in a bowl and apply on clean skin. Leave on for 20 minutes, and then rinse off with tepid water.

Coffee & Cocoa Antioxidant Mask
(not for those with rosacea)

Ingredients:
2 tbsp. fresh ground coffee
1 tsp. organic cocoa powder
2 tbsp. cream

Combine ingredients and apply on clean skin. Leave on for 20 minutes. Rinse with tepid water.

Coffee Face Firmer & Skin Brightener (not for those with rosacea)

This face and neck tightening mask provides a mini facelift and brightens uneven skin tones. Coffee contains over 400 antioxidants and minerals that protect your body from free radicals - some of which include vitamins A1, B1, B2, C, D, E, calcium, magnesium, iron, potassium, zinc, copper, phosphorus and chromium to name a few. When applied topically, the antioxidants in coffee can do wonders for the skin.

Ingredients:
4 tbsp. fresh, cool coffee grounds
1 tbsp. cream
1 tbsp. plain yogurt
1 egg white

Combine all ingredients. Apply on clean face and neck. Leave on 20 minutes, then rinse off.

Calming & Brightening Mask

Ingredients:
3 tbsp. cooked oatmeal
1 tbsp. honey
2 tbsp. cream

Mix all ingredients and apply on face, neck and hands. Wait 20 minutes and rinse off.

Butternut Squash Mask

Butternut squash contains antioxidants, minerals and vitamins that are essential for healthy, beautiful skin. Rich in carotene and vitamins A and C, this mask brightens and firms aging skin.

Ingredients:
⅓ cup mashed cooked acorn squash
2 tbsp. olive oil
1 tbsp. ground almond meal

Combine ingredients and apply on clean skin. Leave on for 20 minutes and then rinse off with tepid water.

Skin Toners

Peppermint Facial Tone
(normal to oily skin)

Ingredients:
2 peppermint tea bags
¼ cup boiled water
2 tbsp. witch hazel
1 drop grapefruit seed extract such as NutriBiotic®

Place the tea bags into the boiled water and steep for 10 minutes. Remove bags and allow tea to cool to room temperature. Add the remaining ingredients, transfer to a BPA-free Glad® storage container and place in the refrigerator. After cleansing skin, apply the toner with a cotton ball. Discard after 10 days and make a fresh batch.

Green & Ginkgo Tea Facial Toner
(dry, mature skin)

Ingredients:
2 organic green tea bags
2 ginkgo tea bags
¼ cup boiled water
2 tbsp. witch hazel
1 drop grapefruit seed extract such as NutriBiotic®

Place the tea bags into the boiled water and steep for 10 minutes. Remove bags and allow tea to cool to room temperature. Add the remaining ingredients, transfer to a BPA-free Glad® storage container and place in the refrigerator. After cleansing skin, apply the toner with a cotton ball. Discard after 10 days and make a fresh batch.

Aloe & Chamomile Tea Facial Toner
(sensitive skin)

Ingredients:
2 organic chamomile tea bags
¼ cup boiled water
1 tbsp. aloe vera
1 tbsp. witch hazel
1 drop grapefruit seed extract such as NutriBiotic®

Place the tea bags into the boiled water and steep for 10 minutes. Remove bags and allow tea to cool to room temperature. Add the remaining ingredients, transfer to a BPA-free Glad® storage container and place in the refrigerator. After cleansing skin, apply the toner with a cotton ball.

Blemishes/Acne & Oily Skin

Blackhead Eliminator

The natural acids in these antioxidant-rich fruits help to gently open pores!

Ingredients:
1 slice tomato
1 slice grapefruit

First, take a slice of tomato and rub it on clogged pores for about 30 seconds. Wait two minutes. Then rub a slice of grapefruit over skin for another 30 seconds. Leave juices on for another five minutes. Then rinse with tepid water. Repeat this regimen three evenings in a row. On night three, you can gently remove the blackheads.

Acne Mask

Turmeric is a spice that can help lighten acne scars and help calm breakouts.

Ingredients:
½ tsp. turmeric powder
1 tsp. olive squalane or food grade coconut oil

Combine turmeric powder with squalane or coconut oil. Before bed time, apply the mixture to clean skin by spot dabbing it on acne or blemish breakouts and old scars using a cotton swab. Leave on overnight. You may also double this recipe and apply to the entire face for skin brightening. Use an old pillow case as turmeric may stain.

Coconut Exfoliating & Hydrating Mask

Though I noted this mask in previous recipe category, it is also beneficial for those with acne or oily skin.

Ingredients:
½ tsp. coconut oil (organic food grade)

Food grade coconut oil rejuvenates and hydrates all skin types, fades wrinkles, sun spots, scars and prevents acne/blemish breakouts! This non-pore-clogging oil gently exfoliates (sloughs off) and strengthens underlying tissues. It's rich in caprylic acid which keeps acne/blemishes in check. Coconut oil absorbs into the skin's cells and helps fight free radical damage associated with sun exposure and keeps blemishes and acne in check.

Use this recipe before bedtime. Run a metal spoon under hot water. While the spoon is still warm, scoop about ½ tsp. coconut oil from the jar onto clean fingertips. The solid coconut oil will easily melt on fingertips as you spread it *sparingly* on clean skin.

Mouth & Lip Recipes

Un-petroleum Jelly Recipe

Ingredients:
½ cup shea butter
6 vitamin E capsules
3 tbsp. olive oil
3 drops rosemary essential oil
2 drops grapefruit seed extract by NutriBiotic® (natural anti-bacterial and preservative)

Melt butter in the microwave. Poke the vitamin E capsules open and add the oil to the melted butter. Add the remaining ingredients and stir well. Pour into Glad® BPA-free plastic storage containers or buy small lip balm-sized metal containers at a craft or beauty supply store and wrap as gifts. Use un-petroleum jelly on lips, chapped hands, neck, feet and under eyes.

Natural Lip Stain

Ingredients:
1 soft toothbrush
1 tsp. baking soda
1 tbsp. water
1 beet
1 clean eye shadow brush

To smooth and prepare the lips, first dip a soft toothbrush in water, then in baking soda and gently brush the lips. Rinse and dry them. Second, cut one slice of beet and set aside. Dip a clean eye shadow brush into water and then rub the wet brush on the beet slice - soaking up the beet juice, and paint the rich, red juice on lips. For a darker shade, wait two minutes for the first coat to dry, and then apply a second coat.

Mouth Line Eliminator

Ingredients:
1 ripe papaya
1 small bottle emu oil

Cut a slice of papaya. Remove the seeds and pulp and rub the inside of the peel over lines around and on lips. Leave on for 20 minutes and rinse with tepid water. Papaya is loaded with nature's retinol so it helps smooth wrinkles. Before bed, apply a drop of emu oil on the area and massage well into skin. Leave on overnight. Emu oil helps thicken and smooth wrinkled or thinning skin in just weeks. Apply papaya two times a week and emu oil nightly.

Mouth Line Smoother & Plumper

Ingredients:
1 tsp. baking soda
1 bottle Hyaluronic Acid Hydrating Mist

Apply baking soda on wet, clean skin in a gentle, circular motion. Focus on the fine lines around the mouth. Rinse with tepid water and apply your day or evening cream or serum. Then spray a little *Hyaluronic Acid Hydrating Mist* on the area. Hyaluronic acid quenches and plumps dry, wrinkled or dehydrated skin. Find the mist in **Safe, Effective Face & Body Product Suggestions**.

Lip Soother

Ingredients:
¼ tsp. honey
½ tsp. vitamin E oil or castor oil

Apply raw, unpasteurized honey on lips and top with vitamin E or castor oil. Leave on overnight. Raw honey helps smooth and heal peeling, chapped lips. Vitamin E heals and moisturizes. Castor oil hydrates and seals in moisture. Leave on lips overnight.

Lip Polisher

Xylitol is a natural sweetener that looks and feels like sugar. Use it to make this effective lip polisher.

Ingredients:
2 tbsp. xylitol (natural sweetener)
1 tsp. food grade coconut oil

Combine xylitol (natural sweetener) with coconut oil to make a paste. Put the paste on a toothbrush and gently scrub lips. Find xylitol at a health food store.

Instant Lip Plumper

Ingredients:
1 hyaluronic acid capsule
¼ tsp. emu oil

Combine the contents of the HA capsule with the oil and massage into lips to stimulate plumpness. Hyaluronic acid (HA) is a moisture magnet. Emu pushes the HA deep down into the lips. As noted throughout this book HA can be applied topically or taken as an oral supplement to effectively hydrate the lips, skin, eyes, and joints. See HA products listed in **Safe, Effective Face & Body Product Suggestions**.

Eye Recipes

Potato Dark Circle Eliminator

Raw potato contains enzymes that help brighten dark under eye circles and the starch helps firm delicate eye skin to reduce puffiness.

Ingredients:
⅓ raw white potato
1 small metal cheese grater

While reclined, apply freshly-grated potato under each eye. Keep eyes closed and take this time to meditate or pray and de-stress. After 30 minutes, remove potato and gentle push the potato juice into the dark circle area. Allow the juice to dry for another 10 minutes. Then rinse with tepid water and dark circles will be lightened. Follow with a moisturizing eye cream. See some powerful choices in **Safe, Effective Face & Body Product Suggestions**.

Grape Skin Puffy Eye Eliminator

Dark grape skins are rich in age-defying resveratrol and vitamins C and E.

Ingredients:
3 chilled black or red grapes

Cool the grapes in the refrigerator for one hour. Then, carefully peel the grapes and <u>save the grape skins</u>. To address eye puffiness, gently dab one of the cooled, peeled <u>skinless</u> grapes under each eye. Then take a reclining position and use a mirror to place the grape skins (wet side down) under each eye. Relax for 20-30 minutes. Rinse with cool water.

Tea Bag Puffy Eye Eliminator

The tannins in green tea reduce eye puffiness.

Ingredients:
2 green tea bags
¼ cup boiled water
4 ice cubes in ½ cup cold water

First, dip tea bags into boiled water to release the anti-inflammatory tannins. Then dip the hot tea bags into ice water. Squeeze water from cooled tea bags and place them on the eyes for 10 minutes.

Eye Hydrator

This eye oil is rich in omega fatty acids for deep hydration.

Ingredients:
1 castor oil capsule or ¼ tsp. castor oil
¼ tsp. squalane oil

Combine the oils and gently press under and around the eyes at night before bed.

Hand Recipes

Hand Scrubber

Ingredients:
½ cup corn meal
2 tbsp. olive oil
1 tbsp. honey

Combine ingredients in a small bowl and stir until they become a paste. Scrub hands for two to three minutes. Rinse and enjoy gorgeous, soft hands!

Invigorating Hand Softener
(this can be used on feet too)

Used coffee grounds can make hands and feet smooth and pretty.

Ingredients:
4 tbsp. used, cool coffee grounds
4 tbsp. salt
2 tbsp. cream
2 tbsp. olive oil
2 drops peppermint essential oil

Combine coffee grounds and salt. Stir in cream and olive oil. Add essential oil, stirring well. Sit on the side of the tub and gently scrub each foot and then scrub hands. Rinse well and pat feet and hands dry. Follow with a hydrating lotion.

Strengthen Brittle Nails

Ingredients:
3 tsp. argan oil
2 tsp. fresh lemon

To help strengthen soft and brittle nails, combine equal parts oil with juice. Dip clean, unpolished nails into the mixture for 10 minutes. Rinse nails and massage with the remaining argan oil. Follow this regimen three times a week. Each night, massage nails with argan oil and wear cotton gloves while you sleep. Do not apply nail polish for one to two weeks.

Carrot Hand Healer

Carrots help hydrate and nourish dry, chapped hands. They are rich in carotene, copper and vitamins C & E.

Ingredients:
2 medium-sized carrots, cooked and mashed
2 tbsp. honey
2 tbsp sour cream
1 tbsp. oats
2 zip lock storage bags (large enough to fit each hand) (**no smaller than 7" x 7½"**)

Combine ingredients in a glass bowl and stir. Divide the mixture into two 7" x 8" storage bags (big enough to fit each hand) and place hands into each bag for 30 minutes. Rinse off with tepid water.

Age Spot Reducer for Hands & Forearms

The scrubbing action of baking soda, the lactic acid in yogurt and bleaching power of lemon juice make this an effective recipe for reducing age spots on hands and forearms.

Ingredients:
6 tbsp. plain yogurt
3 tbsp. fresh lemon juice
10 -12 tbsp. baking soda
1 tsp. olive oil

Combine yogurt, lemon juice and baking soda to make a paste. Scrub the paste on tops of hands and the forearms for 2 minutes. Then, leave the mixture on hands and arms for 20 minutes. Rinse off with tepid water. Afterward apply olive oil or your favorite moisturizer on skin.

Anti-Fungal Nail Soak

Below is a natural anti-fungal nail soak recipe.

Ingredients:
6 oz. fresh ginger
4-5 pieces Chinese licorice root
4 cups water

Mash the licorice root and ginger using a mallet and place in a pot containing the water. Bring to a boil for 5 minutes. Let cool slightly, then strain. Soak fingers or feet in the warm, tea-colored water for 15 to 20 minutes, then towel dry.

Dry Cuticle & Brittle Nail Banisher

Ingredients:
3 tbsp. orange juice
6 tbsp. buttermilk or yogurt

Combine the ingredients in a medium-sized bowl and soak fingers in mixture for 10 minutes. Rinse and dry hands. Rub olive oil into cuticles and nails to keep them moist. TIP: Apply oil nightly and leave on overnight.

Body Recipes

Body Exfoliating Coffee Scrub

Used coffee grounds help smooth away dry, dead skin cells, and improve circulation. Olive oil is a carrier and salt is a preservative that sloughs off dead skin.

Ingredients:
1 cup used, cool coffee grounds
½ cup sea salt
½ cup olive oil

Combine ingredients to form a thick paste-like scrub and store in a plastic food storage container. While in the shower, grab a handful of scrub and in a gentle, circular motion, massage it onto legs, arms, chest, and even knees and elbows. Rinse and then pat skin dry. Use this recipe 3-4 times weekly.

Invigorating Body Scrub

Ingredients:
1 cup granulated sea salt
¼ cup almond oil
10 drops peppermint essential oil

Mix ingredients together in a Glad® BPA-free plastic storage container. After showering, apply the body scrub on wet, clean skin in a gentle, circular motion. Rinse skin and pat dry. Use this recipe 3 - 4 times weekly.

Sun Burn Soother

To prevent a sun burn, re-apply sunscreen every 2 hours whenever outdoors. In the event of a sun burn, this recipe can help soothe skin.

Ingredients:
3 green tea bags
3 tbsp. aloe vera
1 cup boiled water
3-5 cotton balls
1 facecloth

Place the tea bags in boiled water. Let steep and cool. Then add aloe vera gel and stir. Smooth the mixture on sunburned face with cotton balls. For larger areas, double the recipe, dip a clean facecloth into the mixture, lightly wring it out, and apply. Leave on for 20 minutes or longer. Aloe vera calms and heals burns and prevents scarring and the tannins in tea are loaded with anti-inflammatory agents that reduce red, inflamed skin.

After Sun Cream

The oils in this super hydrating rejuvenator can provide many benefits. Shea butter is an ideal moisturizer for all skin types. Coconut oil hydrates and calms inflammation while it attacks free radicals from sun damage. It strengthens underlying tissues, provides elasticity, and helps reduce spots and lines caused by sun exposure. Both coconut and emu oil contain antibacterial properties making them ideal for oily skin too. Safflower oil mimics the skin's natural oils.

Ingredients:
½ cup shea butter
¼ cup coconut oil (food grade)
5 tbsp. emu oil or safflower oil

Place shea butter and coconut oil in a glass bowl and melt in a microwave or double-boiler. Add oil and stir. Pour into a BPA-free storage container and let cool to room temperature. Apply the rejuvenating, non-pore-clogging hydrator to body and face.

Knee & Elbow Scrub

Ground walnuts, corn meal and yogurt make an excellent skin exfoliant and brightener. Lactic acid in yogurt brightens and loosens trapped pores and walnuts exfoliate and hydrate skin.

Ingredients:
2 tbsp. ground walnuts
2 tbsp. corn meal
2 tbsp. yogurt
1 tbsp. honey

Combine ingredients and massage onto clean skin in a gentle circular motion for two minutes per area. Rinse with warm water.

Stretch Mark Repair Recipe

NOTE: Do not use if pregnant as this recipe contains potent essential oils that penetrate deep into the skin. For use after pregnancy only.

Ingredients:
1 small jar (1.7 oz.) of shea butter
1 tsp. lemongrass essential oil
3 tbsp. emu oil
1 capsule evening primrose oil or vitamin E

Heat shea butter in the microwave (remove the cap first). Add lemongrass essential oil and emu oil. Puncture one capsule of evening primrose or vitamin E oil and add to mixture. Stir ingredients and pour into BPA-free Glad® storage container. Apply to stretch marks three times daily. Helps fade red/blue stretch marks and can help tighten skin on tummy. Recipe can be used on old or new stretch marks.

Model's Secret Weight Reduction Bath

Ingredients:
8 oz. hydrogen peroxide
½ carton Epsom® salts (approx. 1 lb.)
Warm to fairly hot bath water

Add peroxide and salts to bath water. Soak for 20 minutes. Afterward, rinse and pat skin dry. You will lose a few pounds and your skin will be silky smooth.

Buchu Tea Weight Eliminator

To sweat out toxins, water weight or to cure what ails you, drink this effective tea about 30 minutes before soaking in the model's secret weight reduction bath (above). Keep a bottle of water by the tub to sip while in the tub. This will prevent dehydration. **Warning**: Do not drink buchu tea more than twice a month! **NOTE**: Consult with your physician before trying this recipe.

Ingredients:
1 dropper full buchu extract
1 cup boiled water

Add a dropper full of buchu extract to a cup of hot water (available at health food stores).

Leg Recipes

Self-Tanner for Legs (and arms)

Instead of sunbathing or using controversial tanning beds, my natural self-tanner recipe gives skin a healthy sun-kissed glow! It does not rub off on your clothes and it stays on until showered off. **NOTE**: This self-tanner recipe will 'stay put' provided you are not dancing, swimming or working up a sweat. It is healthy for skin too. Cocoa is loaded with sun-protecting anti-oxidants and tea provides an excellent tanning shade and anti-inflammatory tannins.

Ingredients:
1 cup water
12 tea bags (Lipton®)
¼ tsp. pure unsweetened cocoa powder

Heat water to boiling; then put 6 of the 12 Lipton® tea bags into the boiled water and steep for 20 minutes. Remove tea bags, making sure to squeeze each tea bag to capture as much of the tint as possible. Then re-boil the steeped tea water and add the remaining 6 Lipton® tea bags to the re-boiled tea water. Again, squeeze each tea bag well when removing them. Add cocoa powder to the hot tea water and stir. Allow the tea water to cool to room temperature. To apply the self-tanner, dip a bristle hair pastry brush into the tea mixture and paint the tanner onto clean legs and arms using long, even paint strokes. Allow the tea to dry for 5-6 minutes before getting dressed.

Clay Mask Cellulite and Toxin Eliminator

Ingredients:
½ cup bentonite or china clay powder
⅓ cup apple cider vinegar
1 med. glass bowl

Mix clay powder with apple cider vinegar in the glass bowl. Find ingredients at a health food store. Apply a thin layer (approximately 1/16") of the mixture to cellulite-prone areas and let dry. Toxins are drawn out as the clay dries. Once dry, gently shower off the clay using a loofah or facecloth.

Pageant Leg Wrap

This recipe is used by many women in beauty pageants to smooth the look of cellulite.

Ingredients:
Preparation H® Cream
Preparation H® Ointment
Cellophane wrap

Combine equal parts Preparation H® cream with Preparation H® ointment and slather onto the noticeable cellulite on the thighs. Wrap thighs with cellophane and leave on for two hours before unveiling. If you have a set of rubber thigh wraps, you may apply those over the cellophane to induce heat. Then remove the cellophane and massage the cream/ointment into thighs. This provides a temporary smoothing effect which lasts for hours.

Spider Vein Reducer

Ingredients:
1 tsp. witch hazel
1 tsp. horsetail herb
2 oz. bottle of emu oil

Combine witch hazel and horsetail and rub mixture on spider vein areas. Apply emu oil on top, massaging into the veins. Natural emu oil is loaded with omega 3, 6 and 9s and is a transdermal oil. Applying it over the active ingredients pushes the solution into the spider veins to help with fading.

Alternate Cellulite Smoother Recipe

Caffeine in coffee constricts blood vessels, temporarily causing skin to appear tighter, firmer, and smoother so it can temporarily reduce the appearance of dimpled skin.

Ingredients:
1 dry brush
½ cup used, caffeinated, warm coffee grounds
1 roll cellophane food wrap
2 sheets of newspaper
1 loofah or facecloth

STEP 1: Dry brush each thigh for 2 minutes before applying the recipe. Dry brushing helps release toxins and boosts circulation. Purchase a dry brush for under $5 at a beauty supply or drug store. While standing on newspaper, apply the coffee grounds to cellulite areas. Most of the grounds will fall to the floor. However, the moist, brownish caffeine and antioxidant-rich residue will be left on skin.

STEP 2: Wrap residue-moistened thighs with cellophane. Wait 40 minutes, remove cellophane, brush any remaining grounds onto the newspaper, then shower, scrubbing the thighs with a loofah or face cloth. The dimple-smoothing effect on thighs lasts for hours.

Foot Recipes

Banish Foot Odor & Swollen Feet

Ingredients:
8 black tea bags
2 cups boiled water
2 cups room temperature or warm water
1 large shallow pail (to fit two adult feet)

Steep tea bags in boiled water. Cool to room temperature and pour tea into a foot bath. Add two cups of plain, warm water. Soak feet 30 minutes. The anti-inflammatory tannins in tea kill bacteria that causes foot odor and reduces swelling.

Oatmeal Foot Softener

Ingredients:
1 cup oatmeal
4 tbsp. lemon or orange juice
4 cups warm water
1 large shallow pail (to fit two adult feet)

Pour the ingredients into the pail and stir until mixed. Soak feet for 20 minutes, then rinse. Your feet will be fabulously soft.

Invigorating Foot Softener
(this can be used on hands too)

Used coffee grounds can make feet smooth and pretty.

Ingredients:
4 tbsp. used, cool coffee grounds
4 tbsp. sugar
2 tbsp. cream
2 tbsp. olive oil
2 drops peppermint essential oil

Combine coffee grounds and sugar. Stir in cream, olive oil and essential oil, stirring well. Sit on the side of the tub and gently scrub each foot. Rinse well and pat feet dry.

Un-petroleum Jelly Recipe

This recipe is noted in several sections because it can be used on many body parts including the feet.

Ingredients:
½ cup shea butter
6 vitamin E capsules
3 tbsp. olive oil
3 drops rosemary essential oil
3 drops grapefruit seed extract (preservative)

Melt shea butter in the microwave. Poke open vitamin E capsules and add oil to melted butter. Then add olive and rosemary oil and grapefruit seed extract (natural antibacterial and preservative) and stir well. Pour into a small Glad® BPA-free plastic storage container and rub onto dry heels after showering or before bedtime. Put on some socks and leave on overnight.

Hair Recipes

Sweet Potato Hair Conditioner

Sweet potatoes are rich in hydrating omega 3 and 6 fatty acids and vitamins A, C and E. This mask conditions and prevents fly away hair. The sweet potato hydrates and nourishes, the honey hydrates and the yogurt removes product buildup and hydrates.

Ingredients:
½ large, cooked, mashed sweet potato
1 tbsp. honey
½ cup plain yogurt

Combine ingredients in a glass bowl and apply to hair. Put on a plastic shower cap, warm a towel in the dryer and wrap it around your head to heat up the hair mask. Leave on for 20 minutes and rinse off with tepid water.

Dry Scalp & Dandruff Relief

Ingredients:
2 peppermint tea bags
½ cup apple cider vinegar
1 cup boiled water
1 BPA-free plastic bottle

For dry, itchy scalp, pour boiled water over two peppermint tea bags and let steep. Add ½ cup apple cider vinegar and let cool to warm temperature. Pour mixture into a plastic bottle and place in your shower stall. Shampoo and condition hair as usual, then use this as a final rinse. Massage it into scalp and leave in hair. Comb out and dry hair. NOTE: Hair will not smell like vinegar.

Scalp Hydrator & Hair Growth Stimulator

A dry scalp can prevent healthy hair growth. Keep the scalp hydrated and nourished with pure rosehip seed oil. It penetrates deep into the scalp and skin.

Ingredients:
2 tbsp. warm rosehip seed oil
1 plastic shower cap

Slightly warm the oil in a small glass bowl in the microwave for 10 seconds. Massage the oil into scalp for five minutes. Put on a plastic shower, warm a towel in the dryer for 5 minutes and wrap it around the head to increase oil penetration. After 1 or 2 hours, remove the cap and shampoo and condition hair as usual.

Hair Hydrator

This recipe addresses dry hair and split ends.

Ingredients:
½ avocado
½ banana
1 tbsp. honey
1 tbsp. olive oil
1 plastic shower cap
1 towel

Combine mashed avocado and mashed banana in a bowl. Add honey and olive oil and mix well. These four super hydrators work synergistically. Massage the mask into hair from scalp down to ends. Put on a plastic shower cap, warm a towel in the clothes dryer for 5 minutes, then wrap around hair. The heat will activate the ingredients. After 30 minutes, rinse out the mask and shampoo hair. Rinse hair with cool water. This helps close the hair follicles, seals in the hydrators and smoothes split ends.

Split Ends Smoother

Ingredients:
¼ avocado
4 drops lavender essential oil
1 small plastic bowl

Mash avocado and add oil. Shampoo hair as usual and apply the hair mask from middle, down to ends of hair. Leave on 20 minutes and rinse with cool water. The combination of the mask and cool rinse closes the follicles, helps seal split ends and makes hair healthy and shiny.

Hair Conditioning Pak

Ingredients:
½ mashed avocado
1 slightly beaten egg
¼ cup olive or safflower oil

Combine avocado, egg and olive or safflower oil. Shampoo hair first and then apply mixture to wet hair. Put on a shower cap and leave on for 30 minutes. To boost penetration, warm a towel in a dryer and cover the shower cap. Do this once a month.

Shiny Hair Rinse

Sea kelp is a fantastic ingredient for shiny hair. It's rich in vitamins and nutrients. This recipe is a quick and effective way to achieve extra shine. Find sea kelp powder at a health food store.

Ingredients:
4-5 tsp. sea kelp powder
2 cups warm water

Add kelp powder to water and stir well until the kelp dissolves. Pour the mixture into a plastic bottle and store in the shower. After shampooing and conditioning hair, pour one cup of the mixture into clean hair. Massage into scalp and throughout hair. Leave in hair for 5 minutes. Rinse and towel dry and you'll be left with super shiny hair.

Brassy Hair Banisher

After swimming in a chlorinated pool, those with red or blonde hair can experience brassy or green-looking hair.

Ingredients:
1 cup cream or whole milk or 1 can of club soda

To banish brassy hair, pour cream or whole milk on hair. Leave on for 10 minutes. Lactic acid in milk helps neutralize the color. Another option is club soda. Pour a bottle of club soda on hair and massage from scalp down to ends. Leave in hair for 10-15 minutes, then rinse with cool water.

Natural Brunette Hair Rinse

Black tea contains tannic acid that can help dark hair look shiny.

Ingredients:
2 black tea bags
2 cups hot water

Place two black tea bags in 2 cups of hot water. Let steep, then cool and remove tea bags. Shampoo and condition hair as you normally do; then use the black tea as a final hair rinse.

Brunette Hair Color Refresher

Coffee enhances brunette hair color and adds shine to hair.

Ingredients:
1 pot of brewed coffee at room temperature
1 plastic bottle

Pour slightly warm coffee into a plastic bottle and store in the shower. First shampoo and rinse hair. Then pour the warm coffee onto clean hair, massaging it well. Put on a plastic shower cap and leave on for 20 minutes. Then rinse with cool water to help seal in the coffee color and close the hair follicles.

Natural Red Hair Rinse

Ingredients:
2 cranberry tea bags
2 cups boiled water
2 tbsp. freshly squeezed lemon juice

For natural redheads, lemon juice and cranberry tea can add highlights to hair. Place tea bags in boiled water with the lemon juice. Let steep, cool and remove tea bags. Shampoo and condition hair as usual, then use this mixture as your final hair rinse. Leave in hair.

Natural Blonde Hair Rinse

Ingredients:
2 chamomile tea bags
2 cups hot water
¼ cup apple cider vinegar

For natural blonde hair, place tea bags in hot water and apple cider vinegar mixture. Let cool and remove tea bags. Shampoo and condition hair as usual, then use mixture as your final rinse. Leave in hair.

Dry Scalp Help for Psoriasis & Eczema

Ingredients:
1 tsp. rosehip seed oil
1 tbsp. jojoba oil

Combine the oils and massage onto scalp, focusing on dry, flaky patches. Leave on overnight. In the morning, shampoo and condition hair with gentle hair products that are free of sodium lauryl sulfates (SLS). See two nice brands in **Safe, Effective Face & Body Product Suggestions**.

Sun Burned Scalp

Ingredients:
1 cup boiling water
2 peppermint tea bags
½ cup apple cider vinegar

Place tea bags and apple cider vinegar into a bowl. Add boiled water. Let cool and place in a BPA-free plastic bottle. Keep the bottle in the shower. Use as a final rinse after shampooing.

Tender Scalp Remedy

For a dry, inflamed or tender scalp, this recipe is very effective.

Ingredients:
2 St. John's Wort tea bags
1 cup hot water

Place 2 St. John's Wort tea bags in water. Let steep and cool to room temperature. St. John's Wort offers anti-inflammatory properties. After shampooing, massage the scalp with tea for 5 minutes. Rinse hair with cool water.

Scalp Clearing Mask for those with natural hair color

Ingredients:
½ papaya
1 shower cap

To help keep scalp clear and prevent product buildup, mash or blend the pulp of ½ papaya and massage into scalp and hair. Put on a shower cap and wait 20 minutes. Then, shampoo and rinse hair as usual.

Oil Treatment for Brittle & Color-Processed Hair, Dandruff or Dry Scalp

Argan oil is an excellent capillary mask for beautiful hair. It nourishes and revitalizes hair, adds lustrous shine, natural softness and silkiness.

Ingredients:
1-2 tbsp. argan oil

Massage argan oil into scalp and hair. Wait at least 30 minutes before shampooing or leave on overnight. For those with flakes, dryness, eczema or psoriasis on the scalp, massage argan oil into scalp and throughout hair at night. Leave on all night, then shampoo in the morning. Argan oil will not stain your pillow case.

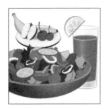

My Favorite Healthy Meal & Snack Recipes

Below are some of my favorite healthy food and beauty recipes. They're easy to make and taste delicious. Many of the recipes are low glycemic or high in fiber, and some are also gluten or flour free. These recipes were created by my husband and me, as well as by my mother. The recipes are large enough for one or two individuals unless otherwise noted. Enjoy!

Breakfast Choices (**Gluten Free)

**Yogurt Bowl

This high protein and fiber breakfast bowl is low glycemic too.

Combine 4 oz. of plain organic yogurt and 1 tsp. fruit-sweetened organic blueberry or raspberry jam and mix together. Then sprinkle 2 tsp. ground flaxseeds, 1 tsp. raw sunflower seeds, raw slivered almonds, or raw walnuts and ¼ cup fresh blueberries or raspberries. Stir and eat. Delicious!

Want more protein? Choose greek style yogurt or stir in ½ scoop of plain whey or soy protein powder into the yogurt and jam. Allergic to dairy? Choose soy or rice yogurt, available at health food stores.

**French Toast & Eggs

For one serving, you'll need 2 egg whites, 2 whole eggs, 1 tsp. ground flaxseeds, 1 tbsp. organic Half & Half® cream, 1 slice gluten and wheat-free bread (see suggestion below), 1 tsp. agave syrup or fruit sweetened jam. I like **Food For Life® Multi-grain Brown Rice Bread** with flax, sesame, pumpkin and sunflower seeds. **NOTE:** Contains millet and rice flour.

Combine egg whites, ground flax and cream. Dip the bread into the mixture. Place the saturated bread in a non-stick frying pan or lightly oil the pan with non-GMO canola or grape seed oil. Cook for two minutes on each side. Then, fry or scramble two eggs and serve them on the side. Top with agave syrup or fruit sweetened jam.

My High Protein, Blueberry & Banana Pancakes (Yields 4 regular pancakes)

100% Flour & Wheat-free Pancakes - Yummy!

These pancakes are loaded with protein and fiber. They are 100% wheat-free and taste absolutely delicious! My husband and I make them on Sunday mornings with two eggs on the side.

STEP 1: Combine ¾ cup ground almond meal, 2 tbsp. ground flaxseeds, 2 tbsp. plain whey or soy protein powder, 1 tbsp. chia seeds, 1 tsp. natural vanilla flavoring, ½ tsp. baking soda, a pinch of salt, 2 eggs, and ¾ cup of buttermilk (or milk of your choice) including soy, almond or rice milk. Mix all ingredients together. NOTE: Add more buttermilk if thinner batter is desired. Thaw 3 tbsp. frozen blueberries and cut ½ banana into slices.

STEP 2: Coat the frying pan with a little grape seed, or non-GMO canola oil and pour enough pancake batter into the HOT pan to make two regular-sized pancakes at one time. Wait one minute, and then add 1 tbsp. thawed frozen blueberries or banana slices onto the cakes. Flip cakes with a spatula after two minutes, and cook for additional 2-3 minutes on other side. Top with maple or agave syrup or fruit-sweetened jam.

**Spinach and Feta Egg White Omelet

Place 4 organic egg whites into a small non-stick frying pan. Cook on one side for 2 to 3 minutes, then flip the whites using a spatula and cook for another minute. Sprinkle 1 tbsp. feta cheese, and a handful of raw, organic spinach onto the cooked egg whites. Fold and serve with a side of hot organic black beans and salsa.

**Cheese and Tomato Egg White Omelet

Place 4 organic egg whites in a small non-stick frying pan. Cook on one side for 2 to 3 minutes, then flip the whites using a spatula and cook for another minute. Drizzle one tbsp. of organic cheddar or swiss cheese, and three slices of organic tomatoes on the cooked egg whites. Fold and serve with hot organic black beans and a little hot sauce on the side.

**Baked High Protein Egg Frittata (Yields 6 slices)

On weekends, when you have more time for breakfast, make a baked egg frittata. Cut into pieces for the week or make it for a family breakfast or get together.

Lightly coat a shallow brownie pan with olive or non-GMO canola oil. In a glass bowl, combine 6 egg whites and 6 whole eggs with ¼ cup milk or Half & Half® cream. Beat this mixture and pour into the brownie pan. Then sprinkle a handful of shredded low-fat mozzarella or white cheddar over the top. Bake at 350 degrees for 18 minutes.

Serve on a slice of toasted protein or rice bread. Spread some Dijon® mustard and Vegenaise®, or olive oil mayonnaise onto the bread, top with a slice of baked frittata and a little salsa if desired. Delicious!

The Ultimate Low Carb High Protein Blueberry Bran Muffins (Yields 6 large muffins)

Once you taste my famous blueberry bran muffin recipe, you'll be hooked! This recipe makes 6 large muffins - big enough to split. And it's low carb and low glycemic! Set the oven temperature to 350 degrees. Grease a large muffin pan with non-GMO canola oil, organic Earth Balance® or coconut oil.

STEP 1: Combine 4 tbsp. Earth Balance® spread, butter or coconut oil with ¼ cup of xylitol (natural sweetener) and blend together with a mixer until creamy. Add 2 eggs, ½ tsp. pure vanilla, 4 tbsp. agave syrup and ¾ cup of organic apple sauce.

STEP 2: In a separate bowl combine the dry ingredients: 1 cup oat bran, ¾ cup ground hazelnut meal or almond meal flour (100% nuts), ¼ cup lentil flour, 2 tbsp. ground flaxseeds, 1 tbsp. chia seeds, ¾ tsp. baking powder, ¼ tsp. baking soda, ½ tsp. sea or himalayan salt and mix together.

STEP 3: Gradually pour the dry ingredients into the wet ingredients and mix together. Once mixed, fold one cup of organic frozen blueberries into the batter. Scoop the mixture into the muffin pan.

Bake for 40 minutes. Prick with a toothpick to ensure they are fully baked. If not, bake for another 5 minutes. Delicious!

Egg Dishes (**Gluten Free)

Prepare two eggs the way you like them (fried, poached, soft boiled, or scrambled) and <u>serve with any one</u> of the following combinations:

**One scoop of low-fat organic cottage cheese, one slice of tomato, avocado, and a side of salsa.

**One piece of turkey bacon and a side of low-fat cottage cheese or ½ cup of warm black beans.

**One slice of toasted gluten-free *Food for Life* rice bread topped with 1 tsp. organic raw almond butter and 1 tsp. fruit-sweetened raspberry or strawberry jam.

Breakfast Protein Shakes (**Gluten Free)

**High Protein & Fiber Breakfast Shake

In a blender combine 1 scoop of whey protein (vanilla or chocolate), 1 tbsp. ground flaxseeds and 1 tsp. chia seeds with 10 oz. of water and 3 ice cubes.

**High Protein & Fruit Breakfast Shake

In a blender combine 1 scoop of vanilla whey protein powder, 1 tbsp. ground flaxseeds, 1 tsp. chia seeds, ⅓ cup frozen blueberries or raspberries and 10 oz. of water.

Lunches & Dinners (**Gluten Free)

---

*Garlic Olive Oil Dressing (GOOD):

This yummy recipe was created by my husband. He has owned and managed several successful restaurants and coffee shops. Use it for salads and on steamed vegetables, steaks, chicken or fish. It's healthy and delicious. Enjoy!

Combine 1 cup of organic cold pressed olive oil with 6 crushed cloves of garlic, the juice of 1 organic lemon, and ⅓ cup of balsamic or apple cider vinegar. Let stand at room temperature for 6 hours. Add sea salt or Himalayan Pink Salt® and black pepper to taste. Then store in the refrigerator. The oil will solidify. When needed, run a metal spoon under hot water or use the gas flame on your stove. Then insert the heated spoon into the cold dressing and remove what you'll need for salads and veggies.

Garlic Olive Oil Dressing (GOOD) serving size TIP:
Drizzle 1-2 tbsp. GOOD dressing on a salad for one.
Drizzle 2-3 tbsp. GOOD dressing on a salad for two.
Drizzle 4-5 tbsp. GOOD dressing on a salad for four.

Salads (**Gluten Free)

**Place 2 cups chopped romaine lettuce or mixed baby field greens in a bowl. Top with two slices of tomato, one sliced boiled egg, 1 tsp. dried organic cranberries, and a scoop of tuna salad. When preparing tuna salad, substitute Vegenaise®, olive oil mayonnaise, or mashed avocado for regular mayo. Pour a little GOOD dressing onto the green salad. See the recipe at the top of this section.

**I love this low-carb chicken caesar salad. Combine a bowl of chopped romaine lettuce, sliced green onions, 1 sliced, hormone-free grilled chicken breast and 1 tbsp. shredded parmesan cheese. Skip the croutons. TIP: Rather than pour dressing on salad, dip your fork into gluten-free caesar dressing before each bite. You'll taste the dressing with every mouthful and eat less fat and calories.

**Combine chopped organic romaine lettuce, organic arugula, diced red onions, and top with a piece of grilled wild salmon. Spread 1 tsp. organic pesto on the salmon and dress the salad with a little *GOOD dressing and salt and pepper to taste.

**Make a seafood salad with chopped romaine, fresh spinach leaves and sliced green onions. Top the salad greens with cooked shrimp or crab, tomatoes and sliced olives. Then top with some *GOOD dressing, salt and pepper to taste, or your choice of healthy salad dressing.

**Make a cobb salad with chopped romaine or field greens, and sliced green onions. Top with a sliced boiled egg, diced turkey breast, diced tomatoes and crumbled blue cheese. Serve with organic ranch dressing or some *GOOD dressing with salt and pepper to taste.

**Make a greek salad with chopped romaine or mixed field greens, black olives, tomato slices, boiled eggs and feta cheese and top with *GOOD dressing and salt and pepper to taste, or your choice of healthy salad dressing.

**To make a southwest salad, chop two cups of romaine lettuce and add some mixed field greens. Add 3 tbsp. pinto and black beans, 2 tbsp. sweet corn, and 1 tbsp. feta cheese. Top with healthy ranch dressing or *GOOD dressing and add sea salt and pepper to taste.

The following three-bean salad is one of my husband's signature salad recipes. It was a hit at his restaurants.

**Combine one 15 oz. can (BPA-free) organic french cut green beans (drained), once 15 oz. can organic pinto and garbanzo beans (drained), 1-2 cloves of fresh garlic (pressed), 1 tbsp. chopped italian parsley, 4 tbsp. fresh lemon juice, 5 tbsp. balsamic vinegar, 1 tsp. Dijon® mustard, 6 tbsp. organic olive oil, sea salt and black pepper to taste. Combine the ingredients in a large bowl, let marinate for 20 minutes, and then refrigerate.

**Salmon

Rub *GOOD dressing on wild salmon, and top with ground pepper and salt. Pan-fry salmon in 1 tbsp. olive oil and serve with steamed asparagus or green beans and a small green salad. Top the veggies with *GOOD dressing or a little pesto sauce.

**Filet Mignon

Rub *GOOD dressing on both sides of the filet, and top with ground pepper and salt. Barbeque the steak and serve with steamed broccoli or artichoke, and a small green salad. Top the broccoli with *GOOD or organic blue cheese dressing.

**Italian Spaghetti Sauce (vegetarian)

My Mom's amazing italian spaghetti sauce recipe is made with 100% veggies. Serve it over quinoa pasta and some healthy, lean meatballs. See my husband's delicious meatball recipe (below).

Combine one onion (quartered), 4-5 tbsp. italian parsley, 6-7 cloves of fresh garlic, 2 celery stalks and 2 medium carrots (cut into one-inch pieces) in a food processor and process until diced into fine pieces. Then heat 2 tbsp. organic olive oil in a large stainless steel pot. When the oil is heated, add the contents of the food processor and stir fry for two to three minutes. Then add two small cans of organic tomato paste and continue to fry the ingredients for three to five minutes. Next add two 15 oz. cans crushed, organic tomatoes and 1 large can peeled, whole organic tomatoes. Add italian seasoning and salt and pepper to taste. Allow sauce to come to a boil and then simmer for 1 hour.

Johnnie's Delicious Italian Meatballs

To make Johnnie's delicious meatballs, combine 1 lb. lean organic beef, 1 egg, 1 tsp. crushed garlic, ½ finely chopped red onion, 1-2 tbsp. chopped italian parsley and a drizzle of hot sauce. Mix the ingredients and form meatballs. Place balls on a cookie sheet and sprinkle each ball with a little shredded parmesan cheese. Bake at 350 degrees for approx.30 minutes. Serve with 1 cup of cooked quinoa pasta, vegetable spaghetti sauce and a small side salad.

Ultimate Meatloaf Recipe

To make Johnnie's meatloaf recipe, follow the meatball recipe (above). Then, add three hot italian chicken or pork sausages, 1 tsp. hot sauce, and 3 tbsp. ketchup. Place in a 5" x 9" glass loaf pan, top with three sliced green olives and bake at 350 degrees for approx. 40 minutes. Serve with a side of steamed green beans or broccoli and a small salad. Top the veggies and salad with *GOOD dressing.

Healthy Fried Chicken or Fish

Make healthy fried chicken, cod or halibut fish by substituting bread crumbs with ground almond meal and use lentil flour instead of regular flour before dipping chicken into egg batter.

STEP 1: Break open two eggs and place them in a big soup bowl. Dip skinless chicken or fish pieces in lentil flour, then into the raw egg bowl, then coat the pieces in almond meal. Add salt, pepper and garlic powder to the 'breaded' chicken or fish.

STEP 2: Fry fish or chicken in fresh olive oil, non-GMO canola or grape seed oil. Serve with a small side salad and one steamed artichoke. NOTE: Discard oil after one use. Never reheat oil as cooling and reheating oil is carcinogenic. This is a good reason to avoid eating fried foods in restaurants.

The Best Split Pea Soup

If you're a fan of split pea soup, you're going to love this recipe.

Chop 1 organic carrot and 1 celery stalk into ¼ inch pieces and place in a bowl. Next place 2 more carrots, 1 onion, 1 stalk of celery, and 3-4 cloves of peeled garlic into a food processor and grind. Heat 1 tbsp. olive oil in a large pot and add the processed veggies, frying for three minutes. Rinse one bag (16 oz.) of organic green split peas and pour over the fried veggies. Then add the diced carrot and celery stalk and cover with 5-6 cups of water or combine 2 cups organic chicken broth and 4 cups water (if you're not a vegetarian) and bring to a boil. Then reduce to simmer for one hour and 20 minutes. Be sure to stir every 20 minutes. Add salt and pepper to taste. It's delicious and full of fiber. Drink lots of water when you eat high fiber foods to prevent bloating.

**Delicious 'Ramen' Soup with Shiritaki Noodles

This guilt-free, carb-free 'Ramen-like' noodle soup is better and healthier than the real thing. It's another one of Johnnie's creations. The noodles are virtually carbohydrate free.

Heat 1 tbsp. olive oil in a large frying pan. Dice ½ onion into fine pieces, slice 6-8 mushrooms and dice ½ zucchini (or any veggies of your choice) and sauté. Rinse one 8 oz. package of shiritaki noodles in a colander. Add the rinsed noodles to the pan and stir-fry them with the veggies for 1 minute. Add 2 cups organic chicken broth. Bring to a boil. Crack two eggs and place into the soup. Place a lid on the pan and allow the eggs to cook for three minutes. Delicious!

**Tasty Bean and Spinach Stew

Johnnie's black bean and spinach stew is outstanding.

Heat 2 tbsp. olive oil in a skillet. Add ¼ cup finely chopped onion and 2 cloves crushed garlic. Sauté onions until transparent. Then add garlic. Cook for 1 minute. Add one 15 oz. can crushed organic tomatoes, one 12 oz. bag of washed organic baby spinach leaves, one 15 oz. can of organic black beans and pinto beans. Add salt and pepper to taste. Cover and simmer for 15 minutes and serve as a side dish or over quinoa or cooked shiritaki noodles.

**Lentils and Quinoa with Salad

This is one of my favorite meals.

STEP 1: Place ½ cup of rinsed organic lentils in a small sauce pan, cover with 1 cup water and cook for 20-30 minutes (until soft). In a second sauce pan cook ¾ cup rinsed quinoa in 1 ½ cups water or organic chicken broth and cook for approximately 15 minutes. Add a little salt to the water. Afterward, drain pans into a colander and set the lentils and quinoa aside.

STEP 2: Pour 2 tbsp. organic olive oil in a skillet and add ½ onion, finely diced. Cook until transparent. Add the cooked lentils and quinoa, salt and cayenne pepper to taste. Fry the mixture for three minutes. Then prepare a mixed green salad with romaine lettuce, chopped tomatoes, green onions, salt and pepper to taste, and *GOOD dressing. To serve, place two scoops of the lentil/quinoa stir fry onto a plate and top with green salad.

**Butternut Squash Recipe

Set oven to 400 degrees. Cut the squash in half (lengthwise), remove the seeds and place both halves cut-side-up on a baking sheet. Brush the tops of both halves with a little olive oil and place into the oven. Cook for 35-45 minutes until soft. Scoop out the cooked squash and eat it as is or mash with a little cinnamon or organic Earth Balance® spread.

Snacks (**Gluten Free)

**Hi-Protein – Low Fat Deviled Eggs (without the yolks)

Egg whites are high in protein and low in calories. One of my favorite snacks is un-deviled eggs.

STEP 1: Boil 6 eggs. To make the perfect boiled egg, place 6 eggs in a small pot, cover with water and turn heat to high. When the water comes to a full boil, turn off the heat and cover the pot. Leave eggs in hot water for 15 minutes. Then drain, let the eggs cool to room temperature, and peel them.

STEP 2: Slice the eggs in half (lengthwise) and scoop out the yolks. Combine two scoops of low-fat cottage cheese or four slices of avocado, with ½ tbsp. Dijon® mustard, and add a sprinkle of paprika, garlic, pepper and salt or Spike® Gourmet Natural Seasoning (all-purpose/salt free) in a blender or food processor until creamy. Spoon the mixture into the hollowed egg whites and enjoy a high protein snack without the fat and cholesterol.

**Healthy, Tasty Hummus Dip

If you like hummus, you're going to love Johnnie's recipe.

Drain 1 can of organic garbanzo beans and pour into a food processor. To this add 3 tbsp. tahini, 4-5 tbsp. organic olive oil, the juice of one whole lemon, 1 clove of crushed garlic, ¼ tsp. of cumin, salt and pepper to taste. For more spice, add a little drizzle of hot sauce. Blend well and gradually add 2-4 tbsp. of water to smooth the consistency. If you desire a thinner consistency add a little more water when blending. Refrigerate to cool and serve with celery, zucchini, cucumber, red peppers, carrot sticks, raw cauliflower or broccoli.

**Greek Yogurt and Cilantro Dip

This tasty dip is high protein and low fat.

Combine 8 oz. of plain greek yogurt, 1 tbsp. finely chopped cilantro, 4 chopped chives, 1 crushed garlic clove, 1 tbsp. olive oil and stir together. Add salt and pepper to taste. Cool in the refrigerator for 30 minutes and serve with raw vegetables instead of corn chips. I like raw celery, zucchini, cucumber, red peppers, carrot sticks, raw cauliflower or broccoli.

**Nuts

Pistachios are one of the lowest caloric nuts. They're rich in antioxidants, fiber, and healthy unsaturated fats. A ¼ cup of unshelled pistachios is about 80 calories, 3 grams of protein, 2 grams of fiber and 7 grams of fat, so they make an excellent heart-healthy snack. Cracking the shells prevents overeating. If watching salt intake, choose unsalted or low-salt versions. Keep nuts stored in the refrigerator. Walnuts and almonds are good choices too. They're loaded with omega 3 fatty acids.

**Edamame Soy Pods

Edamame soybean pods make a delicious, healthy snack. Boil the pods for 5 minutes and top with a sprinkle of sea salt, or not. Soy pods are high in protein and fiber, essential fatty acids, soy isoflavones and low in fat.

Crispbread with Healthy Toppings

Crispbread comes in a variety of flavors. My favorite is Ryvita® sesame rye. One slice is only 40 calories, 4 grams of fiber, zero trans fats and it's made with three ingredients; whole grain rye, sesame seeds and salt. These crackers are quite large so you'll need only one.

Place any of the following toppings onto one slice of Ryvita®:
-1 slice of organic goat cheese and 2 sardines (packed in olive oil)
-1 scoop of tuna or chicken salad
-1 slice of baked turkey or chicken breast with red pepper and hummus
-2 slices of tomato with a drizzle of *GOOD dressing and shaved parmesan cheese on top. Eat this cold or place into a toaster oven.

Avocado on Toast

Toast a slice of sprouted protein bread or Food for Life® Rice Bread. Then top with a thin slice of Gouda® goat cheese and two slices of avocado for a delicious, satisfying snack.

**Olive & Turkey Wrap

Olives are loaded with healthy plant-based omega 9 fatty acids. Snacking on olives is one of Sophia Loren's tips for beautiful skin.

Slice 4 to 5 green or black olives. Roll the olive slices and a leaf of romaine lettuce in a thin slice of baked turkey or chicken.

**Roasted Garbanzo Beans (AKA Chickpeas)

Roasted garbanzo beans make an excellent high fiber snack.

Heat the oven to 400 degrees. Drain one 15 oz. can of organic beans and place into a bowl. Add 2 cloves of crushed garlic, 2 tbsp. organic olive oil, salt, and pepper and mix well. Place foil wrap on a baking sheet and spread the coated beans evenly on the sheet. Bake for 30 minutes or until crunchy.

**Johnnie's Kale Chips

You'll need a food dehydrator for this kale chip recipe. Dehydrating foods at 115 degrees help maintain their enzymes and nutrients. Kale is a super food that is rich in over 45 flavonoids, antioxidants, omega 3 fatty acids and more. Read more nutritional benefits of kale in **Age-Proofing Tip #53 - Super Foods.**

STEP 1: Combine ½ organic red pepper, ¾ cup raw organic cashew pieces, 1 cup non-GMO and gluten-free nutritional yeast, 1 tbsp. fresh lemon juice, 1 tsp. chia seeds, ½ tsp. salt, ½ tsp. pepper, 1 crushed clove of garlic and blend in a food processor to make a thick paste-like consistency.

STEP 2: Wash one large bunch of organic kale. Remove the veins and stems, chop kale into two inch pieces and place in a large bowl. With clean hands, coat the leaves with the paste.

STEP 3: Place the coated leaves on the dehydrator tiers, and sprinkle each layer with a little himalayan sea salt. Set the dehydrator to 115 degrees. Wait 5 hours and check crispness of kale chips. If not yet crisp, dehydrate for one more hour. Once kale is crisp, transfer the chips into a glass or BPA-free plastic storage container with a paper towel over the top, then seal. The paper towel will absorb any moisture. Eat the kale chips within 2-3 days as they spoil quickly.

**Apple & Nut Butter

Scoop 1 tbsp. of almond, or combination almond/flax butter onto a plate. Slice half an organic apple into bite-sized slices. Then dip slices into the nut butter for a high protein and fiber snack that's low-glycemic.

**Sugar-free Chia Pudding

Chia seeds are packed with fiber, protein, and heart healthy plant-based omega 3 and 6. Just 1 tbsp. contains contain 6 grams of fiber and 3 grams of protein.

Combine ¼ cup chia seeds with one cup of soy, rice, almond or coconut milk, and 2-3 tbsp. organic cocoa powder. Sweeten with 3 tbsp. xylitol or ½ tsp. organic stevia and stir. Chill in the refrigerator for three hours.

**Apple Bake

Finely slice two apples and sprinkle 2 tsp. xylitol, or a little stevia, 1 tbsp. fresh lemon juice, a pinch of salt and mix together. Place in a loaf pan and bake at 350 degrees for 30 minutes. Serve with cold yogurt on top. This is a delicious low calorie treat.

Chocolate Tofu Pudding & Berries (4-5 servings)

You'll love this dairy and sugar-free pudding, made with chocolate and tofu. It's easy to make and tastes divine!

Melt 6 oz. dark chocolate and 4 tbsp. xylitol or 1 tsp. stevia in a microwave or double boiler over medium heat to melt the chocolate. Combine melted chocolate, 6 oz. soft silken tofu, and ¼ cup water in a food processor, add a pinch of salt, and blend until smooth. Place in the refrigerator and chill for one hour. To serve, place chocolate tofu pudding into bowls and top with fresh raspberries and blueberries.

High Protein & Fiber/Low Carb Bread Recipe (6 servings)

This bread recipe does not rise too high and is a little spongy, but it is tasty. I use this recipe to make gluten-free toast and spread almond butter and fruit-sweetened raspberry jam on it. It's also great for French toast.

STEP 1: Heat oven to 350 degrees. Lightly grease an 8" x 8" loaf pan with a little Earth Balance® Whipped Organic Buttery Spread. In a separate bowl, beat 6 egg whites until stiff and set aside. Save the yolks.

STEP 2: In a larger bowl, combine the yellow egg yolks, ¼ cup soy flour, ¼ cup ground almond meal, ¼ cup ground flaxseeds (AKA flax meal), 6 tbsp. of hormone-free plain yogurt or sour cream, 5 tbsp. of Earth Balance® (or butter), 2 tbsp. fresh baking powder and beat together.

STEP 3: Fold the egg whites into the contents of the large bowl, and transfer all into the loaf pan. Bake for approximately 45 to 50 minutes at 350 degrees. Use a toothpick to check if bread is completely baked.

**Protein Bars

Quest Bars® are one of the most delicious protein bars that I have eaten to date. They are 100% natural, free of artificial sweeteners or sugar alcohols, they are gluten-free, high fiber and offer 20 grams of protein and 4 or more grams of fiber. My two favorite flavors are Coconut/Cashew™ and Lemon Cream Pie™. They are naturally sweetened with stevia, a 100% natural, zero calorie sweetener. Find Quest bars at many health food stores in the USA.

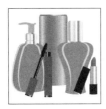

Safe, Effective Face & Body Product Suggestions/Resources

As you have read, facial and body products can affect our health, hormones, weight, mood and well-being. Switch to healthy products that are free of parabens, synthetic fragrances (phthalates), petroleum and synthetic dyes. Be an ingredients 'sleuth'. Read all product labels.

NOTE: The products noted below and throughout this book are known to be free of harmful ingredients. However, be sure to read all labels or contact the manufacturers to confirm ingredients prior to use. Use the products at your own risk.

For product sources CHECK the legend below which notes where to find specific products noted throughout this book. If you do not have access to some of the retailers noted below, you can purchase several items at cost-effective prices at www.HollywoodBeautySecrets.com. They are noted as *HBS.

NOTE: Some products are subject to change due to availability. Prices may be subject to change.

Product Source Legend

Available at HollywoodBeautySecrets.com at discount prices **(*HBS)**
Available at Health Food Stores **(HFS)**
Available at Drug Stores **(DS)**
Available at Grocery Stores **(GS)**
Available at Beauty Supply Stores **(BS)**
Available at Bed, Bath & Beyond **(BBB)**
Available at Doctor's offices **(DO)**
Available at Select Spas **(SS)**
Unless otherwise noted

Facial Cleansers
-Glycolic Cleanser with Marina Plant Extracts (Mature, dry skin) ***HBS, HFS**
-Reviva® Labs Glycolic Acid Cleanser **HFS**
-DMAE/Alpha Lipoic/C-Ester Cleanser (For body too) ***HBS, HFS**
-Beyond Clean (With salicylic acid for oily skin) ***HBS, DO, SS**

Facial Toners
-Anti-Aging Pycnogenol Toner (For all skin types) ***HBS, HFS**
-Vitamin A Glycolic Toner **HFS**
-Soy & Papaya Toner **HFS**

Facial Exfoliators (Scrubs & Creams)
-Microdermabrasion Scrub (Exfoliant) ***HBS, HFS, BBB**
-Evenly Radiant Overnight Peel (AHA cream moisturizing exfoliant) ***HBS, HFS**
-Glycolic Cleanser with Marina Plant Extracts (Exfoliating cleanser) ***HBS, HFS, DS, BBB**
-Beyond Clean (Salicylic acid exfoliating cleanser) ***HBS, DO, SS**
-Baking Soda **GS**
-Papaya **GS**
-Lemons **GS**
-Plain dairy or soy yogurt **GS**

Sunscreen
-Evenly Radiant Day Crème 15 SPF (Face & body) ***HBS, HFS**
-Aubrey Organics Natural Sun SPF30 Green Tea Sunscreen (Face & body) **HFS**
-Devita® Natural Skin Care Solar Protective Moisturizer SPF 30+ **HFS**
-Sunology® Crème for Face **BBB, HFS**
-Neutrogena® Pure & Free Liquid Daily Sun Block SPF 50 (Face & body) **DS, BBB**
-Johnson & Johnson® Baby Daily Face & Body Lotion, SPF 40 **DS**

EGF Creams (Epidermal Growth Factors For Face & Neck)
For Mature, Normal or Menopausal Skin that needs more volume:
-Ultimate Age-Proofing Complex (EGF, peptides & antioxidants for day or night) ***HBS, DO, SS**
For Mature, Sensitive, Dry or Menopausal Skin that needs more volume & hydration:
-De-Aging Solution (EGF, squalane, HA & antioxidants for day or night) ***HBS, DO, SS**

Peptides (Face, neck, décolletage, and tops of hands)
-Night Perfect Serum (100% peptides in glycerin base) ***HBS, DO**
-Uplift Serum (Peptides, antioxidants & HA for day or night) ***HBS, DO**
-MyChelle® Polypeptides Cream **HFS**
-Beyond Essential (Peptides & antioxidants for oily skin for day or night) ***HBS, DO**
-Deep Penetrating LED Peptide Serum (Use with LED Red Light) ***HBS, SS, DO**
(See peptide eye creams in the eye section)

Copper Peptides (acne, broken capillaries)
-Beyond CP ***HBS, DO, SS**

Antioxidants (Face, Neck, Décolletage, Hands)
-Age-Defying Night Crème (Astaxanthin® & Pycnogenol®) ***HBS, HFS**
-Evenly Radiant Night Crème® (Skin brighteners that fade spots) ***HBS, HFS, BBB**
-Wrinkle Reduction (Antioxidants with emu oil & glycolic acid for night) ***HBS, DO, SS**
-DMAE/Alpha Lipoic/C-Ester Crème (AKA Firming Moisturizer) **DS, HFS,***HBS**
-MyChelle® Vitamin A Serum **HFS**
-Avalon® Organics Vitamin C Renewal **DS, HFS**
-Simple® Hydrating Light Moisturizer **DS**

272

Pycnogenol® Products
-Age-Defying Night Crème (Astaxanthin® & Pycnogenol®) *HBS, HFS
-Pycnogenol® supplements HFS

Hyaluronic Acid Products (Hydration for Face & body)
-Hyaluronic Hydrating Mist (HA & antioxidants - apply under moisturizer & set makeup) *HBS
-De-Aging Solution (EGF cream with HA, squalane & antioxidants) *HBS, DO, SS
-Ultimate Age-Proofing Complex (EFG, HA, antioxidants & peptides) *HBS, DO, SS
-Evenly Radiant Night Crème (Skin brighteners & HA) *HBS, HFS, BBB
-Skinlasting Super Hydrator (HA, vitamin C, green tea for neck & body) *HBS, DS, DO
-Uplift Serum (Peptides, antioxidants & HA for face, neck & body) *HBS, DO
-Beyond Essential (Peptides, antioxidants & HA for oily skin) *HBS, DO, SS
-Refill Wrinkle Filler *HBS, DO, SS
-Deep Penetrating LED Serum (Peptides & HA) Use with LED Red Light or emu oil *HBS, DA, SS
-Country Life®Hyaluronic Acid supplements (80 ml) HFS

Creams with Pomegranate Seed & Rosehip Oil
-Ultimate Age-Proofing Complex *HBS, DO, SS
-Beyond Essential *HBS, DO, SS
-Beyond CP *HBS, DO, SS

Emu Oil Products
-Emu oil 100% pure *HBS, HFS
-Emu lip balms (3 pack) *HBS, HFS
-Ultimate Eye Crème *HBS, SS, DO
-Wrinkle Repair (Peptide & antioxidant-rich night cream)*HBS, DO, SS

Squalane Oil Products
-100% pure Squalane oil (Derived from olives) *HBS, HFS
-De-Aging Solution (EGF, squalane & antioxidants) *HBS, DO, SS

Beauty Oils
-100% Emu oil *HBS, select HFS
-100% Squalane oil (From olives - not sharks) *HBS, Select HFS
-100% Rosehip seed oil *HBS, HFS
-100% Coconut oil (Food grade) HFS
-100% Argan oil *HBS, HFS
-100% Jojoba oil HFS
-Pomegranate seed oil HFS

Neck Lifting Help
-Evenly Radiant Overnight Peel with AHA (Moisturizing exfoliant) *HBS, HFS
-De-Aging Solution (EGF cream, squalane, HA & antioxidants) *HBS, DO
-Ultimate Age-Proofing Complex (EGF cream, peptides & antioxidants) *HBS, DO
-Night Perfect Serum (Peptides in glycerin base) *HBS, DO, SS
-Uplift Serum (Peptides & antioxidants water-based serum) Day or night *HBS, DO, SS
-Evenly Radiant Day Crème *HBS, HFS, BBB
-Skinlasting Super Hydrator (Apply under moisturizer) *HBS, DS, DO
-Hyaluronic Hydrating Mist *HBS, HFS
-LED Red Light Therapy DO, SS, *HBS (best price on the web)
-Deep Penetrating LED Serum *HBS, SS
-Skinnies ™ Instant Lifts (Cut to size) instantlifts.com
-Water-proof bandages DS

Eyes, Lashes & Brows
-Baby pink under brow hi-lighting pencil *HBS, Sephora®
-RapidLash® Eyelash & Eyebrow Enhancing Serum *HBS, DS, BBB,
-Argan oil *HBS, HFS
-Define-A-Brow™ (brow pencil) DS, GS
-Brow Wiz by Anastasia® (brow pencil) Sephora®
-Brow Sculpting Marker® laurageller.com
-Black eye liner pencil Wet 'n' Wild® DS
-White eye liner pencil Wet 'n' Wild® DS
-Eyelash curler by Revlon® DS
-Lancôme® Paris Definicils High Definition Mascara Sephora®
-Emu oil *HBS, HFS
-Castor oil HFS, DS
-Eye Perfect (trace parabens) *HBS, DO, SS
-Ultimate Eye Crème *HBS, HFS, DO, SS
-Nature's Gate Eye Cream HFS
-Discount prescription & sun glasses GlassesUSA.com
-Polarized sun glasses GlassesUSA.com
-Pinhole glasses DS, Dr. Leonard's Catalogue
-Chamomile & green tea bags GS, HFS
-Astaxanthin supplements HFS
-Hyaluronic acid supplements HFS

Teeth, Lips & Breath
-Sonicare® (Tooth cleaning system) Costco® Target®
-Baking soda DS, GS, Costco®
-Probiotics HFS
-Tom's of Maine® natural toothpaste HFS, DS, BBB
-Nature's Gate® Crème de Peppermint natural toothpaste BBB, HFS
-Oral grade peroxide DS, HFS
-Glide® dental floss DS Costco®
-Crest 3D Whitestrips® with Advanced Seal DS
-XyloSweet® xylitol (Natural sweetener) HFS
-Cinnamon Spry® (Natural xylitol gum) HFS
-Licorice XyliChew®(Natural xylitol gum) HFS
-Cuticle scissor by Revlon® DS
-Magnifying mirror DS, BS
-Lipton® black tea bags GS, DS
-Raw honey HFS
-Vitamin E HFS
-Aveeno® Active Natural Lip Conditioner DS, GS
-Emu Lip Balm (100% natural) *HBS, HFS
-Aubrey Organic® Naturals Moisturizing Lip Gloss *HBS, HFS
-Bert's Bees® Natural Lip Gloss DS, HFS
-Waxelene® (Natural petroleum-free jelly) BBB, HFS
-Chlorella Nutricology.com
-Green tea HFS, GS
-Peppermint tea HFS, GS
-Fennel seeds GS
-SinuCleanse® Neti Pot HFS, DS
-Simply Saline® Arm & Hammer DS
-Ocean® sinus cleanser DS
-Distilled water GS, DS, HFS
-Oil of oregano HFS
-NutriBiotics® Grape Seed Extract HFS
-Quercetin HFS

274

Lip Plumper
-Night Perfect Serum ***HBS, DO, SS**
-Emu oil ***HBS, HFS**
-LED Red Light Therapy *HBS guaranteed lowest price
-Deep Penetrating LED Peptide Serum ***HBS, DO, SS**

Mouth Lines
-Ultimate Age-Proofing Complex ***HBS, DO, SS**
-De-Aging Solution ***HBS, DO, SS**
-Uplift Serum ***HBS, DO, SS**
-Night Perfect Serum ***HBS, DO, SS**
-Hyaluronic acid supplements **HFS**
-Hyaluronic Hydrating Mist ***HBS**, **HFS**
-Emu oil ***HBS, HFS**
-Led Red Light Therapy ***HBS**
-Deep Penetrating LED Serum (For use with LED Red Light) ***HBS, DO, SS**

Canker Sores
-Rescue Remedy® by Bach, **HFS**
-Plain yogurt GS, **HFS**
-Chamomile tea bags **HFS, GS**
-Natura Nectar® Propolis **HFS**
-Y.S. Eco Bee Farms® Propolis **HFS**

Cold Sore Prevention & Relief
-Rescue Remedy® **HFS**
-Dry-brush (Natural bristles) **HFS, BS, DS**
-Garlic capsules Kyolic® **HFS**
-Vitamin D3 **HFS**
-Vitamin C Ester **HFS**
-Olive leaf extract **HFS**
-Grape seed extract **HFS**
-Zymessence® systemic enzymes **solutionstoaging.com**
-Vitalzyme X® systemic enzymes (For vegans & vegetarians) **Check Web**
-Flaxseed oil **HFS**
-Turmeric **HFS, GS**
-Olive Gold 03® **solutionstoaging.com,** ***HBS**
-King Chlorella **Nutricology.com**
-Lavender essential oil **HFS**
-Tea tree oil **HFS, DS**
-Echinacea Supreme Gaia Herbs® **HFS**

Rejuvenating Gadgets that Really Work!
-LED Red Light Therapy (Best price guaranteed) ***HBS**
-Micro-current - Serious Skin Care® **Costco®**
-Derma Rollers **Check the web for many sources**

Topical Product for use with Led Red Light Therapy
-Deep Penetrating Led Serum (Light driven peptides with HA) ***HBS, SS, DO**

Topical Products to use with Micro-current
-Uplift Serum ***HBO, DO, SS**
-Night Perfect Serum ***HBS, DO, SS**
-Aloe vera gel **HFS, DS**
-Microdermabrasion Scrub ***HBS, HFS, SS**

-De-Aging Solution (EGF, HA, antioxidants - sensitive, dry mature skin) ***HBS, DO, SS**
-Ultimate Age-Proofing Complex (EGF, peptides, HA & antioxidants - normal to oily) ***HBS, DO, SS**

Topical Products to use with Derma Rollers
-Night Perfect Serum ***HBS, DO, SS**
-Uplift Serum ***HBS, DO, SS**
-Vitamin C serum **HFS, BBB**

Botox on a Budget
-Uplift Serum ***HBS, DO, SS**
-Refill Wrinkle Filler ***HBS, DO, SS**
-Hyaluronic Acid Hydrating Mist ***HBS, HFS, BBB**
-Deep Penetrating LED Serum ***HBS, DO, SS**
-LED Red Light Therapy ***HBS** best price guaranteed

Winter Wrinkle-Buster AM Protocol
-Glycolic Cleanser with Marine Plant Extracts ***HBS, HFS, DS**
-Anti-Aging Pycnogenol Toner ***HBS, HFS**
-De-Aging Solution (EGF) ***HBS, DO, SS**
-Ultimate Age-Proofing Complex (EGF) ***HBS, DO, SS**
-Hyaluronic Hydrating Mist ***HBS, HFS**
-Uplift Serum ***HBS, SS**
-Evenly Radiant Day Crème (SPF 15 sunscreen & skin brighteners) ***HBS, HFS**

Winter Wrinkle-Buster PM Protocol
-Uplift Serum ***HBS, DO, SS**
-Night Perfect Serum ***HBS, DO, SS**
-Age-Defying Night Crème (Astaxanthin® & Pycnogenol®) ***HBS, SS**
-Emu oil ***HBS, HFS**
-Squalane oil ***HBS, HFS**
-Coconut oil (food grade) **HFS**

Oily Skin/Acne
-Beyond Essential (Day or evening peptide lotion) ***HBS, DO, SS**
-Microdermabrasion Scrub **HFS, *HBS**
-Beyond Clean (Salicylic acid for oily skin) ***HBS, DO, SS**
-Anti-Aging Pycnogenol Toner ***HBS, HFS**
-Vitamin A Glycolic Toner **HFS**
-Beyond CP (Peptides & copper peptides for oily, mature skin) ***HBS, DO, SS**
-O24U Hyperoxygenated Gel (Acne spot treatment & weekly mask) ***HBS, DO, SS**
-Argan Oil (Night treatment) ***HBS, HFS, DS**
-Squalane Oil (Under moisturizer hydrator) ***HBS, HFS**
-Milk Of Magnesia **DS, GS**
-L'Oreal® Studio Effects (Makeup primer) **DS**

Back Acne
-Evenly Radiant Overnight Peel (AHA) ***HBS, HFS**
-Plain yogurt **HFS, GS**
-Plain canned organic pumpkin **HFS**
-Zinc **HFS**
-Vitamin D **HFS**
-Chlorella **Nutricology.com**
-O24U Hyperoxygenated Gel (spot treatment, weekly mask) ***HBS, SS, DO**

Younger-Looking Makeup Needs
-Emu oil **HBS, HBS**
-Ultimate Age-Proofing Complex *****HBS, DO, SS**
-Beyond Essential *****HBS, DO, SS**
-Even Radiant Day Crème (SPF 15 sunscreen & skin brighteners) *****HBS, HFS**
-Boots No. 7® Radiant Glow (Concealer) **Target®**
-Erase Rewind by Maybelline® (Concealer) **DS**
-Laura Geller's Spackle® (Makeup primer) **Laurageller.com**
-L'Oreal® Studio Effects (Makeup primer) DS put in acne skin section
-Foundation brush **Sephora®**
-Baby pink under brow highlighting pencil *****HBS**
-White eye liner pencil by Wet 'n' Wild® **DS, BS**
-Lancome® Paris Definicils High Definition Mascara **Sephora®, Dept. Stores**
-Hair curler roller papers **Sally's Beauty Supply**
-Natural Lips by Aubrey Organics *****HBS, HFS**
-Bert's Bees® Super Shiny Natural Lip Gloss **DS, HFS**
-Aubrey Organics Natural Lips (Gloss) *****HBS, HFS**
-Hyaluronic Hydrating Mist (Dewy finish/sets makeup) *****HBS, HFS**
-Baby wipes by Seventh Generation® (Handy makeup remover) **HFS, BBB**
For brow products see Eyes, Lashes and Brows section.

Mineral Makeup
-Aubrey Organics® Silken Earth **HFS**
-Jane Iredale® **SS, DO, Janeiredale.com**
-Dash® contact Shelly@mineralperfections.com
-Liquid Foundation (organic) contact Bryansawchuk@gmail.com

Deodorant
-Aubrey®E Plus High C Natural roll-on deodorant (Women, men & teens) **HFS**
-Crystal Rock® Deodorant Spray **DS, HFS**
-Tom's of Maine® Deodorant (Stick) **HFS, DS**

Self-Tanners
-Tan Tone (Vitiligo camouflage) **Call 1-877-568-4727 to special order, DO, SS**
-Bronzing Custard Gradual Tanner by Vani-T® (Check Beauty News) *****HBS site**

Sun Spots & Hyper-pigmentation
-Glycolic Cleanser with Marine Plant Extracts *****HBS, HFS, DS**
-Evenly Radiant Day Crème with SPF 15 (Sunscreen) **HFS, *HBS**
-DMAE/Alpha Lipoic/C-Ester Crème *****HBS, HFS, BBB**
-Alpha lipoic acid cream **HFS**
-Evenly Radiant Night Crème **HFS, *HBS**
-Evenly Radiant Overnight Peel (AHA) **HFS, *HBS**
-Skin Lighten **HFS, *HBS, BBB**
-Vitamin C-ester serum **HFS**
-Aubrey Organics Natural Sun 30+ **HFS**
-Neutrogena® Pure & Free Liquid Daily Sun Block **DS**
-Uplift Serum (Peptides, HA & antioxidants) *****HBS, DO, SS**
-Night Perfect (Peptides) *****HBS, DO, SS**
-Beyond Essential (Peptides & antioxidants) *****HBS, DO, SS**
-Microdermabrasion Scrub **HFS, *HBS**
-Camocare® C-Spot **HFS**
-Witch hazel **DS**
-Retin A® (prescription) **DS**
-Evenly Radiant Overnight Peel (AHA) *****HBS, HFS, BBB**

-Pycnogenol® supplements **HFS**
-LED Red Light Therapy *****HBS**
-Coconut oil **HFS**
-Multani mati **Indian GS**
-Turmeric (Spice) **GS, HFS**

Hands

-Anti-Aging Hand Crème (For hands & feet) *****HBS, HFS**
-Evenly Radiant Overnight Peel (AHA cream) *****HBS, HFS**
-Chapstick® (natural formulation) **DS, GS**
-Emu Lip Balm (100% natural) *****HBS, DS**
-LED Red Light Therapy (Lowest price guaranteed) *****HBS**
-Perfect Formula Pink Gel Coat **Sephora®**
-Revlon® Crazy Shine Nail Buffer **DS**
-Almond or olive oil **HFS**
-Orange wood stick **BS**
-Tea Tree oil **HFS**
-Grapefruit seed Extract by NutriBiotic® **HFS**
-Vick's® Vapor Rub **DS**
-Buffing block for nails **DS, BS**
-Four-way nail file **DS, BS**
-Distilled white vinegar **GS**
-Cotton balls **DS, BS**
-Organic nail polish **HFS, Zoya.com, PritiNYC.com**
-Zim's® Crack Crème *****HBS, DS**
-Skinlasting Super Hydrator (For hands, feet & body) *****HBS, DO, SS**
-Country Life® Maxi-Hair Biotin (Growth supplement for nails and hair) **HFS**

Feet

-Omega 3 flaxseed oil supplements **HFS**
-Zim's Crack Crème *****HBS, DS**
-Cortizone-10® **Target®, DS**
-Cocoa Butter **DS, HFS**
-Shea Butter **DS, HFS**

Legs

-Dry Brush **BS, BBB, HFS**
-Morton® Salt **GS**
-Sea salt **GS, HFS**
-Almond oil **HFS, BS**
-Olive oil **GS, HFS**
-Glad® storage containers (BPA-Free plastic) **GS**
-Evenly Radiant Overnight Peel *****HBS, HFS**
-Skinlasting Super Hydrator (HA) *****HBS, DS, SS**
-Uplift Serum (Peptides & HA) *****HBS, SS, DO**
-Hydrating Hyaluronic Acid Mist *****HBS, HFS**
-Shea butter **BS, HFS**
-Lemongrass essential oil **HFS**
-Emu oil *****HBS, HFS**
-Bentonite or china clay **BS, HFS**
-Organic apple cider vinegar **HFS, GS**
-Almond oil **BS, HFS**
-Olive oil **GS, HFS**
-Lipton® (100% natural tea bags) **GS, DS**
-Tan Toner (Self-Tanner with peptides & antioxidants) *****HBS, DO, SS**
-Vani-T® Bronzing Custard (Self-tanner) **Vani-T.com**

-Aubrey Organic Silken Earth Body Shimmer **HFS**
-Horse chestnut (Tincture) **HFS**
-Witch hazel **DS, HFS**
-Arnica gel or cream **HFS**

For Body (Shower or Bath)
-Jason® Natural Body Wash **HFS, DS**
-DMAE/Alpha Lipoic/C-Ester Cleanser (Facial or body cleanser) *****HBS, HFS**
-Nature's Gate® Oatmeal Liquid Soap **HFS**
-Burt's Bees Peppermint & Rosemary Body Wash
-Burt's Bees® Milk & Shea Butter Body Wash **HFS, DS**
-Avalon® Organics **HFS, DS**
-Everyone® Soap **HFS, BBB**
-GentleNaturals™ Eczema Relief Wash (For adults with dry skin) **BBB**
-Organic apple cider vinegar **HFS, GS**
-Green tea bags **GS, HFS**
-Chamomile tea bags **GS, HFS**
-Unsweetened coconut milk **GS, HFS**
-Epsom® salts **DS, HFS**
-Dried lavender **HFS, BS**
-Jojoba oil **HFS, BS**
-Himalayan pink salt **GS, Gourmet Shops**
-Lavender essential oil **HFS**
-Quaker® Oatmeal **GS, DS**
-Dried sage leaves **GS, HFS**
-Dried rosemary **GS, HFS**
-Lemongrass essential oil **HFS**
-Fennel essential oil **HFS**
-Unsweetened coconut milk **HFS**
-Eucalyptus oil **HFS**
-Thyme essential oil **HFS**
-Espom® salts **DS, HFS**
-Jojoba oil **HFS**
-Peppermint essential oil **HFS**
-Rosemary essential oil **HFS**
-Rosehip seed oil *****HBS**
-Nutribiotic® Grapefruit Seed Extract **HFS**
-Distilled vodka **GS, DS**
-Food grade coconut oil **HFS**
-Safflower oil **HFS**
-Glad® storage containers (BPA-free) **GS**
-Shea butter **HFS, BS**
-Earth Therapeutics® Palm brush **HFS, BBB**
-FIR infrared sauna blankets **HollywoodBeautySecrets.com**
-FIR infrared saunas (stand up) **SaunaRay.Com**
-Thermo Green Tea *****HBS, HFS**

Natural Fragrance Oils
-Kuumba Made® **HFS**

Scars, Stretch Marks & Burns
-Derma Rollers **Skinmedix.com**
-Microdermabrasion Scrub (Scars & stretch marks or older burn scars) *****HBS, HFS**
-Earth Therapeutics® Palm brush (dry brushing) **HFS, BBB**
-Rosehip Seed Oil *HBS, HFS
-Scar Gel (Scars, stretch marks & older burn scars) Apply 3 x daily *****HBS, HFS**

-Emu Oil (Scar & stretch mark moisturizer / helps thicken skin) ***HBS, HFS**
-Night Perfect (Peptides that stimulate collagen) ***HBS, DO, SS**
-Uplift Serum (Peptides that stimulate collagen) ***HBS, DO, SS**
-LED Red Light Therapy (Prevents scarring) ***HBS, DO, SS**

Rosacea
-Beyond Clean Cleanser ***HBS, DO**
-Glycolic Cleanser with Marine Plant Extracts ***HBS, HFS**
-Pycnogenal® Gel **HFS**
-Squalane Oil ***HBS, HFS**
-Sea Buckthorn Oil **HFS**
-Argan Oil **HFS,** ***HBS**
-Green tea bags **GS, HFS**
-Age-Defying Night Crème (Astaxanthin® & Pycnogenol®) ***HBS, HFS**
-Alpha Lipoic Creme with Green Tea Complex **HFS, BBB**
-Zinc and vitamin A supplements **HFS**
-Olive Gold 03 **HFS,** ***HBS, solutionstoaging.com**
-Natura Nectar® Propolis **HFS**
-Y.S. Eco Bee Farms® Propolis **HFS**
-Mineral Makeup (see makeup)**HFS**
-Turmeric **GS, HFS**
-LED Red Light Therapy System (best price on web) ***HBS**

Eczema
-Rescue Remedy® by Bach (oral spray) **HFS**
-Borage oil **HFS**
-Rosehip seed oil **HFS**
-Flaxseed oil capsules and flaxseeds **HFS**
-Bee pollen **HFS**
-Honey **HFS**
-Natura Nectar® Propolis **HFS**
-Y.S. Eco Bee Farms® Propolis **HFS**
-B12 Cream **Compounding Pharmacy, HFS**
-Milk Thistle **HFS**
-5-HTP **HFS**
-Chamomile tea **HFS**
-Vitamin E **HFS**
-Vitamin B3 **HFS**
-Ginseng extract **HFS**
-Echinacea **HFS**
-Witch hazel **DS, HFS**
-Hydrocortisone cream **DS**
-Beyond Clean Cleanser ***HBS, DO, SS**
-BabyGanics® Eczema Care Cream (For adults with dry skin) **BBB**
-GentleNaturals™ Eczema Relief Wash (For adults with dry skin) **BBB**
-Olive Gold 03 ***HBS**
-King Chlorella® **Nutricology.com**
-Zymessence™ Systemic Enzymes **SolutionsToAging.com**

Psoriasis
-Beyond Clean Cleanser ***HBS**
-Flaxseed, Flax-Primrose or borage oil combo **HFS**
-Emu oil ***HBS, HFS**
-Borage oil **HFS**
-Oil of oregano **HFS**
-Echinacea **HFS**

-Sea buckthorn oil **HFS**
-Rosehip seed oil **HFS**
-Natura Nectar® Propolis **HFS**
-Y.S. Eco Bee Farms® Propolis **HFS**
-Argan oil *__HBS, HFS__
-B12 cream *compounding Pharmacy*
-Coconut oil *__HBS__
-Vitamin C-ester **HFS**
-Olive Gold 03 **SolutionsToAging.com**
-Zymessence™ Systemic Enzymes **SolutionsToAging.com**
-Milk thistle **HFS**
-5-HTP **HFS**

Keratosis Pilaris
-Microdermabrasion Scrub *__HBS, HFS__
-Beyond Clean (Salicylic acid cleanser) *__HBS, DO, SS__
-Glycolic Facial Wash with Marine Plant Extracts **HFS**, *__HBS__
-Reviva® Labs Glycolic Acid Cleanser **HFS**
-Retin A **DO, DS**
-Evenly Radiant Overnight Peel with AHA **HFS**, *__HBS__, **BBB**
-Skinlasting Hydrating Mist *__HBS, SS, DO__
-Derma E® Refining Vitamin A & Green Tea Crème **HFS**

Vitiligo & Self Tanners
-Tan Toner (Self-tanner with peptides & antioxidants)*__HBS, DO, SS__
-Bronzing Custard (Self-tanner) **Vani-T.com**
-Lipton's (100% natural tea bags) **GS, DS**

Milia
-Microdermabrasion Scrub *__HBS, HFS__
-Evenly Radiant Overnight Peel (AHA cream) *__HBS, HFS__
-Beyond Clean (AHA cream) *__HBS, DO, SS__
-Glycolic Cleanser with Marine plant extracts **HBS, HFS**
-Retin A **DO**
-LED Red Light Therapy **hollywoodbeautysecrets.com**
-Neosporin® (Topical antibiotic ointment or cream)**DS**
-Honey **HFS, GS**

Joint Relief
-Astaxanthin® supplements **HFS**
-Hyaluronic acid supplements by Country Life® **HFS**
-Krill oil supplements **HFS**
-Joint Relief® by Schiff (HA, Astaxanthin® & krill oil) **Costco®**
-Pycnogenol® supplements **HFS, Trader Joes®,**
-Dr. Schulze® Cayenne Powder Blend **herbdoc.com**
-Vitamin C **HFS**
-Vitamin D **HFS**
-Resveratrol **advancedbionutritionals.com**
-FIR infrared sauna blankets **HollywoodBeautySecrets.com**
-FIR infrared saunas **SaunaRay.Com**

Hormone Health
-Whey powder **HFS**
-Flaxseed oil **HFS**
-Evening primrose oil **HFS**

-Vitamin B5 (pantothenic acid) **HFS**
-Vitamin B6 **HFS**
-Vitamin D **HFS**
-Calcium citrate supplements **HFS**
-Magnesium supplements **HFS**
-Chlorella **Nutricology.com**
-Buffered vitamin C **HFS**
-5-HTP Natrol® Tryptophan **HFS**
-Melatonin **HFS**
-Meditropin® **Nutraceutics.com**
-Rescue Remedy® **HFS**
-Squalane oil *****HBS, HFS**
-Hyaluronic acid supplements (Skin & joint hydration) **HFS**
-Supplements **NewChapter.com, ClearMedicine.com, LifeExtension.com**
-FIR infrared sauna blankets *****HBS**
-Body vibration plates *****HBS**
-Organic hemp protein powder **HFS, Nutiva.com, NavitasNaturals.com**

Body Hydrators
-Skinlasting Super Hydrator (For neck & body) *****HBS, DO, SS**
-Hyaluronic Hydrating Mist (For face, neck & body - sets makeup too) *****HBS, HFS**
-Argan oil (Dry skin, eczema, psoriasis) *****HBS, HFS, DS**
-Squalane oil (Derived from olives for all skin types) *****HBS, select HFS**
-BabyGanics® Eczema Care Cream (For adults with dry skin) **BBB**

For Hair
-Your Crown & Glory® Shampoo & Conditioner (For thin, falling hair) *****HBS, HFS**
-Giovanni ® Root 66™ Max Volume Shampoo and Conditioner (Limp hair) **BBB**
-Jason® Shampoo **HFS, DS**
-Nature's Gate® (Shampoo & Conditioner) **HFS**
-Natural Missst Herbal Hairspray -Regular Hold *****HBS, HFS**
-L.A. Hold® Hair Spritz **BBB, HFS**
-LaMaur® VitaE Ultra Hold Professional Spray (Unscented) **Beauty Supply**
-Moroccan Argan Oil (For hair, dandruff, eczema or psoriasis on scalp) *****HBS, HFS**
-King Chlorella **AdvancedBionutritionals.com**
-Arm & Hammer® baking soda (Dry shampoo alternative) **GS, Costco®**
-Kingsford's Corn Starch® (For teasing & dry shampoo) **GS**
-Bob's Red Mill Organic Coconut Flour **HFS**
-Giovanni Powder Power® Dry Shampoo **HFS, BBB**
-King Chlorella® supplement (For shiny hair) **Nutricology.com**
-Country Life® Maxi-Hair Biotin (Hair growth supplement) **HFS**
-Rosehip Seed Oil *****HBS, HFS**
-Sea kelp powder **HFS**
-Coconut flour **HFS**

Supplements
Supplements noted throughout the book are available at health foods stores. I've noted a few of my favorite brands below.
-Hyaluronic acid supplements (80 mg) by Country Life® **HFS**
-Pycnogenol® antioxidant supplements by Country Life® **HFS**
-Ascorbic Acid crystals by KAL® **HFS**
-Ascorbyl Palmitate by Source Naturals® **HFS**
-Advanced EFA's Plant-based Omega 3s & 6s **AdvancedBionutritionals.com**
-Kyolic® Aged Garlic Extract (odorless capsules) **HFS**
-King Chlorella® **NutriCology.com**
-Zymessence™ Systemic Enzymes **SolutionsToAging.com**

-Trans-Resveratrol **HFS, AdvancedBionutritionals.com**
-Zenbev Natural Tryptophan **HFS, Zenbev.com**
-Natrol® 5-HTP (Tryptophan) **Costco®, HFS**
-Genuine Health® whey protein **GenuineHealth.com, HFS**
-Beveri™ whey protein **HFS**
-Dream Water® **GS, Bristol Farms, DrinkDreamWater.com**
-Sam-E **HFS, Costco®**
-Also visit **NewChapter.com, ClearMedicine.com**

Weight Loss
-Kyolic® Aged Garlic (Odorless capsules) **HFS**
-Organic apple cider vinegar **HFS, GS, Trader Joe's Stores**
-Thermo Green® (Green tea capsules) *****HBS, HFS**
-Fat Burner Blast Off Coffee (Blended organic coffee & green tea) *****HBS**
-Natural Organic Raw Green Bush Tea **The Republic of Tea®**
-Dandelion Tea **HFS**
-Organic Stevia Extract **Trader Joes®**
-Windmill's Green Coffee Bean Extract (Caplets) **GNC® stores**
-Bob's Red Mill (Nut flours: coconut, almond meal, hazelnut meal, garbanzo bean) **HFS**
-House Foods® Tofu Shirataki noodles **Asian markets & select grocery stores**
-Shirataki Noodles **Asian markets & select grocery stores**
-Food for Life® Rice Bread **Trader Joes®, HFS**
-Meditropin® (powder packets) **Nutraceutics.com**
-Tantric Toning DVD **StephaniesSacredSelfCare.com**
-Under 30-Minute Model Sculpting Video **HollywoodBeautySecrets.com**
-FIR infrared sauna blankets **HollywoodBeautySecrets.com**
-FIR infrared saunas (stand up) **SaunaRay.com**
-Organic hemp protein powder **HFS, Nutiva.com, NavitasNaturals.com**

Probiotics & Vaginal Health
-Culturelle® Probiotics **DS**
-Candidase® Probiotics **HFS**
-Trunature® Probiotics **DS, Costco®**
-Ultimate Flora® Ultra Protect **HFS**
-BV Essentials® Vaginal Inserts (Homeopathic BV treatment) **HFS, Select DS**
-YeastGuard® Advanced (Homeopathic vaginal suppositories) **HFS, Select DS**

LED Red Light Therapy
HollywoodBeautySecrets.com
-Deep Penetrating LED Serum (Light driven peptides) *****HBS, SS, DO**

Facial Gadgets:
-LED Red Light Therapy **HollywoodBeautySecrets.com**
-Serious Skin Care® (micro-current) **Costco®**
-Facemaster® (micro-current) **Facemaster.com**
-Facial Flex® **Sears.com, *HBS**

FIR Infrared Blankets, Vibration Plates & More
-FIR infrared sauna blankets **HollywoodBeautySecrets.com**
-FIR infrared (stand-up saunas - assembly required) **SaunaRay.com, Activeforever.com**
-Body vibration plates **HollywoodBeautySecrets.com** (wholesale)
-Aero® Pilates home reformer **QVC.com, Target ®**
-Air Climber® **Target®**

Other
-Baking Soda **GS, DS, Costco**
-Dry brush Earth Therapeutic® Body Brush **BBB, HFS**
-Powdered ascorbic acid HFS
-Rescue Remedy® **HFS**
-Meditropin® **Nutraceutics.com**
-Derma Rollers **Skinmedix.com**
-FIR infrared sauna blankets *****HBS**
-LED Red Light Therapy (Best web price) *****HBS**
-Body vibration plates (Best web price) *****HBS**
-Bob's Red Mill® flours (Almond, coconut, hazelnut, garbanzo) **HFS**
-Organic Stevia Extract **Trader Joes®**

Hand Wipes
-Seventh Generation® Free & Clear (Baby wipes) **HFS, BBB**
-BabyGanics® Thick n' Kleen (Face, hand & baby wipes) **BBB**
-Heinz distilled white vinegar **GS**
-Ziploc® sandwich bags **GS**

Doctor and Professional Testimonials:

"If you are in search of **the** *natural beauty expert, look no further. Louisa Graves is truly the ultimate expert in this field. For years, Louisa has been teaching us healthy ways to be beautiful with a knowledge and expertise that are world class. Her teachings are based on non-invasive ways we can both feel and look our best. The way we feel about ourselves matters and with the lessons and suggestions that she presents in* **"Age-Proof: Beauty Alternatives You Need to Know."** *Louisa helps us with improving our self-image challenges."*

Dr. Robert Puff, Ph.D., Clinical Psychologist,
Speaker, Author, Newport Beach, CA

"As a physician and avid listener to Doctor Radio on Sirius XM Radio, one of the most informative and enlightening shows is the Dermatology Show with Dr. Doris Day. I had the good fortune of catching Dr. Day's show with Louisa Graves as the guest expert. Sharing the stage with Dr. Day is a distinction in itself. But it is clear that Louisa's range of expertise is equal with that of many well-respected and knowledgeable practitioners in dermatologic skin care. I see Louisa as an indispensible partner to the doctor's work. Louisa's advice on beauty and age proofing is state of the art, accessible and sensible. I love the idea that Louisa can take natural everyday ingredients as well as scientific findings and blend them together for a unique range of non-invasive beauty and age proofing techniques. Medical professionals and the discriminating individual will find a wealth of well researched information, advice, and products when consulting with Louisa."

Diana Tang, M.D., San Francisco, CA

"I have been a true skin care junkie most of my life, always looking for the latest and greatest product or tool offering that "WOW" result! I admit, when it comes to assessing skin care products, I am a staunch, "tough as nails" critic who might possibly be looking for the impossible; some unrealistic result. I say this because in 20 plus years of an exhausting search, which includes more than a dozen at-home skincare machines/gadgets/tools, hundreds of prescription and dermatologist recommended products, sold only in the most exclusive shops and catalogues, in-office peels and 100s of other products from internet companies and consumer topics on threads like makeupalley.com, I have NEVER found that "WOW" result!!!

That all changed when I came across a website that peaked my curiosity. I placed a phone call to inquire about some of the products, expecting to leave a message. Little did I know that this call would be my 'magic' moment - the one that would end my search and change my life...forever!!! I was met with the warmest, most informative, most sincere, passionate and scientifically sound explanation to every one of my questions...... by the skin care GURU herself, Louisa Graves!! I was so completely absorbed in every last detail of her beauty tips and advice, frantically writing down every spoken word. I have no doubt that Louisa was born with this passion; that inherent in her genes is this love and commitment to her work!!!! She is so current in her knowledge, able to warmly embrace and clearly articulate the answer to each of my questions. She is hands down more competent than any professional with whom I have ever consulted!

I conclude this testimonial with the most valuable information with which I can provide. If you are looking for significant, visible improvement of your skin, if you are skeptical or been frustrated by products that did not deliver, please look no further! I urge you to check out the products listed at HollywoodBeautySecrets.com. I have just emptied out closets of my past purchases, mourning the loss of the hard earned money I wasted on the failed promises from so called "skin care experts."... I have currently tried several of the products recommended at Louisa's website. After 20 years of failed products, I kid you not, my skin is completely transformed! I am truly elated!! That "WOW" result I had been searching for...I now experience it everyday! These amazing products meet every one of my highest, and once thought to be, unrealistic expectations. More specifically, my skin is thicker, tighter, smoother, has a more even skin tone with a glow that visibly radiates! Finally, I must share that each conversation I have had with Louisa Graves only validates and solidifies her professional expertise and wealth of scientific knowledge. She is a true gift in this overwhelming and confusing skincare market."

Dr. Cathy Markle, Assistant Clinical Professor,
Yale University School of Medicine

"Louisa's advice has been keeping me young and fresh for years and she's the first expert I consult whenever I need beauty and health information. Not only is the information in **"Age-Proof: Beauty Alternatives You Need to Know"** cutting edge, but it could actually save your life! Louisa shares how we can uplift and rejuvenate ourselves at reasonable prices and even reveals beauty recipes we can whip up ourselves, at home, with common pantry ingredients. Louisa positively glows from the inside out, graciously sharing her wisdom and research with us all. If you only buy one beauty book, this should be it."

Lisa Johnson Mandell, Journalist, Hollywood, CA
Author of "Career Comeback" and "How to Snare a Millionaire NOW"

"Louisa was a <u>great</u> guest expert on **Sirius Doctor Radio** on **The Dermatology Show with Dr. Doris Day**. Louisa really clicked with Dr. Day – they were 'on the same page' with each topic, sharing very interesting conversations. Louisa was most impressive handling caller questions with Dr. Day. We will have her back as a guest beauty expert again."

Jenna Strolla, Producer
Doctor Radio, Sirius 114/XM 119, NY

Acknowledgements

A number of amazing individuals helped make this book possible. I have much gratitude to those who have mentored and supported me. They include:

My husband John Graves; thank you for helping me run my business, overseeing our household, as well as the many shoulder rubs and nourishing meals you prepared for me each and every day. You make every day feel like Valentine's.

My family; thank you Mom and Dad, for being my role models and for teaching me that a strong work ethic, eating fresh, home-cooked food, and keeping life simple enhances our health and wellbeing. I also thank my sisters Angela, Sonia and Patsy, my brother Daniel, and my sisters and brothers-in law for their love and support. Though you all live thousands of miles away, I know you are close by in my heart. I am blessed by your love and support.

My cover designers; thank you Hunter Business Forms Inc. Print and Promotion; for creating my beautiful book cover design.

My publisher, editors, fact checkers and proof-readers; thank you to Melissa and Ryan Levesque, Blake Boulerice, Anna Cody, Donna Rolen, for your patience and attention to detail.

My illustrator; thank you ShannonCodyDesign.com for creating the illustrations for my book.

My photographer; thank you Babak Delafraz for shooting my beautiful cover shots.

My makeup artist; thank you Maria Nguyen for my fresh and natural-looking makeup.

My hair stylist; thank you Mary Jo Lorei for creating my perfect shade of blonde.

My publicist, Barbara Adolph at NationalPRPros; thank you for believing in me, and for your wisdom and friendship.

All my friends, clients and customers who believe in my mission; I truly thank you for your support, love and sharing your suggestions with me.

All the product developers and manufacturers; though I cannot name you all, thank you for listening to my suggestions and making changes to your products to make them effective and safe for us all.

All the professionals, mentors, colleagues, and contributors; to list everyone would require more space than is available, though I would like to make a special mention; Dr. Alicia Stanton, Dr. Evelynne Llorente, Dr. Robert Puff, Dr. Cathy Markle, Dr. William Wong, Dr. Liu, Dr. Robert Rowen, Dr. Linda Miles, Manuela Stoerzer-Vogt, Lisa Johnson-Mandell, Edward Menster, Isabelle VonOffel, Stephanie DePhillipo, Richard Carieri, Stuart Spangenberg, Aubrey Hampton, Florence Shinn, and Emmett Fox. Thank you for sharing your knowledge and insight with the world.

Empowerment Gal

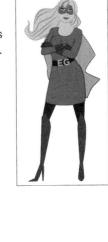

Refer to this book to help get through those times when you need pampering and encouragement. Keep the following in mind.

*You are responsible for your own happiness
and health
Take time for you
Nourish yourself with healthy food
Love yourself
Begin each day with a positive attitude
Create good vibrations
Banish negative thoughts
You have much to offer
You are worthy and strong
Have compassion
See good in others
Be grateful for what you have, your health, family and friends
Keep life simple, enjoy the little things
Do what you love
As you achieve success - give back
Let go of resentment
Forgive
Open your heart to great possibilities
Take pride in all you do
Don't let anyone stand in your way.
You can accomplish what you desire!*

Louisa ☺

If you have an iPhone or an iPad2 or newer, please scan my App on the back cover of this book.

About The Author
Louisa on TV, Radio, the Web & More

Louisa Graves is one of the nation's leading media beauty experts. She has shared her age-proofing tips on myriad television shows and networks including: *The Talk, The Doctors, Extra, The Discovery Channel, The Style Network*, and on morning news shows including *KTLA Morning News* and *KCAL News* in Los Angeles, and more. She has also been a guest expert on 100s of radio shows including: *Sirius XM Doctor Radio, KIIS-FM, WGN-Chicago, Hot97-NewYork, The WAVE, K-EARTH Los Angeles, The John Tesh Network* and many more. Louisa is the author of popular, doctor-recommended book, *"Hollywood Beauty Secrets: Remedies to the Rescue."*

Her tips have appeared in national magazines including *First for Women* and *Woman's World* as well as in newsletters, blogs, documentary films, and popular websites *MSNBC.com, AOLHealth.com, AOLJobs.com, WomansDay.com*, and *SheKnows.com*, just to name a few. She wrote the "Look and Feel Good" series for *AOL/Huffington Post Group* and is a featured panelist for *Ask America's Ultimate Expert* in *Woman's World magazine.*

To date, hundreds of thousands of individuals have viewed her free beauty videos at www.YouTube.com/user/BeautyGuru/videos. For more age-proofing information, visit www.HollywoodBeautySecrets.com and subscribe to her free monthly newsletter. If you have an iphone® or ipad®, access Louisa's app, noted on the back cover of this book. Follow her on www.facebook.com/Hollywood.Beauty.Secrets or www.twitter.com/AgeproofingGuru.